Communicating Prognosis

Core Principles of Acute Neurology

Recognizing Brain Injury
Providing Acute Care
Handling Difficult Situations

Communicating Prognosis

EELCO F. M. WIJDICKS, M.D., PH.D., FNCS, FANA

Professor of Neurology, Mayo Clinic College of Medicine

Chair, Division of Critical Care Neurology

Consultant, Neurosciences Intensive Care Unit

Saint Marys Hospital

Mayo Clinic, Rochester, Minnesota

OXFORD

UNIVERSITY PRESS

OXFORD
UNIVERSITY PRESS

Oxford University Press is a department of the University of Oxford.
It furthers the University's objective of excellence in research, scholarship,
and education by publishing worldwide.

Oxford   New York
Auckland   Cape Town   Dar es Salaam   Hong Kong   Karachi
Kuala Lumpur   Madrid   Melbourne   Mexico City   Nairobi
New Delhi   Shanghai   Taipei   Toronto

With offices in
Argentina   Austria   Brazil   Chile   Czech Republic   France   Greece
Guatemala   Hungary   Italy   Japan   Poland   Portugal   Singapore
South Korea   Switzerland   Thailand   Turkey   Ukraine   Vietnam

Oxford is a registered trademark of Oxford University Press
in the UK and certain other countries.

Published in the United States of America by
Oxford University Press
198 Madison Avenue, New York, NY 10016

Library of Congress Cataloging–in–Publication Data
Wijdicks, Eelco F. M., 1954- author.
Communicating prognosis / Eelco F.M. Wijdicks.
   p. ; cm.—(Core principles of acute neurology)
Includes bibliographical references.
ISBN 978-0-19-992878-1 (alk. paper)
I. Title.   II. Series: Core principles of acute neurology.
[DNLM: 1. Brain Diseases—diagnosis.   2. Neurologic Manifestations.   3. Palliative Care.
4. Professional-Family Relations.   5. Referral and Consultation. WL 141]
RC348
616.8′075014—dc23
2013036371

The science of medicine is a rapidly changing field. As new research and clinical experience broaden
our knowledge, changes in treatment and drug therapy occur. The author and publisher of this
work have checked with sources believed to be reliable in their efforts to provide information that
is accurate and complete, and in accordance with the standards accepted at the time of publication.
However, in light of the possibility of human error or changes in the practice of medicine, neither
the author, nor the publisher, nor any other party who has been involved in the preparation or
publication of this work warrants that the information contained herein is in every respect accurate
or complete. Readers are encouraged to confirm the information contained herein with other
reliable sources, and are strongly advised to check the product information sheet provided by the
pharmaceutical company for each drug they plan to administer.

9 8 7 6 5 4 3 2 1
Printed in the United States of America
on acid-free paper

For Barbara, Coen, and Marilou

Contents

Preface

Any physician needs to know the clinical course of a disorder well enough to know the outcome. This is reasonably established in many major medical disorders and also in neurology. However, knowledge about the outcome of acute brain injury is relatively recent. Not until the 1980s did systematic studies appear on prognosis of coma. Neurosurgical databases of traumatic brain injury were developed to refine the outcome categories. Statistical models have been developed in traumatic brain injury and other major causes of acute brain injury, but much is lacking. Moreover, these models only function if the clinical data entered is reliable and relevant.

Physicians asked to prognosticate—and we all are asked frequently—have a difficult task. Families are involved more than ever before in decision-making, but it is difficult for them to grasp the meaning of percentages. Many think they can beat those odds. In many situations it is the seasoned clinician versus a probabilistic model, and it is not always certain who wins.

I would be disingenuous to say that prognosis of neurologic disorders is intrinsically unknowable. How do we assemble information? Why are we so uncertain in some cases and certain in others? How often and why do patients unexpectedly do well? When can we reliably diagnose a persistent vegetative state? These common questions, and others, are addressed in this volume.

Patients admitted to Neurosciences Intensive Care Units are severely injured and expected to leave with a disability; some will not awaken from coma. With increasing technology—and success in more than a few instances—comes a "we will prevail" attitude. Physicians are motivated to go on, families definitely are, and compromise is rarely on their minds.

How do we define futility, and what do we need to know? What is black, and what is gray? How do we tell the patient's family? What is our proper demeanor? How do we proceed with family conferences, and what are our responsibilities?

These are the other issues discussed in this volume and is mostly centered on palliative care in acutely ill neurologic patients. The family conference raises the delicate matter of how to decide that outcome is indefinitely poor or how to define disability. Separate chapters expose what these the ordeals mean for families and deconstruct physician and nursing staff compassion and describe its most important elements. I hope this book provides straightforward, commonsensical, advice and touches on all aspects of supporting devastated families.

Introduction to the Series

The confrontation with an acutely ill neurologic patient is quite an unsettling situation for physicians, but all will have to master how to manage the patient at presentation, how to shepherd the unstable patient to an intensive care unit, and how to take charge. To do that aptly, knowledge of the principles of management is needed. Books on the clinical practice of acute, emergency, and critical care neurology have appeared, but none have yet treated the fundamentals in depth.

Core Principles of Acute Neurology is a series of short volumes that handles topics not found in sufficient detail elsewhere. The books focus precisely on those areas that require a good working knowledge. These are: the consequences of acute neurologic diseases, medical care in all its aspects and relatedness with the injured brain, difficult decisions in complex situations. Because the practice involves devastatingly injured patients, there is a separate volume on prognostication and neuropalliation. Other volumes are planned in the future.

The series has unique features. I hope to contextualize basic science with clinical practice in a readable narrative with a light touch and without wielding the jargon of this field. The ten chapters in each volume try to spell out in the clearest terms how things work. The text is divided into a description of principles followed by its relevance to practice—keeping it to the bare essentials. There are boxes inserted into the text with quick reminders ("By the Way") and useful percentages carefully researched and vetted for accuracy ("By the Numbers"). Drawings are used to illustrate mechanisms and pathophysiology.

These books cannot cover an entire field, but brevity and economy allows a focus on one topic at a time. Gone are the days of large, doorstop tomes with many words on paper but with little practical value. This series is therefore characterized by simplicity—in a good sense—and it is acute and critical care neurology at the core, not encyclopedic but representative. I hope it supplements clinical curricula or comprehensive textbooks.

The audience is primarily neurologists and neurointensivists, neurosurgeons, fellows, and residents. Neurointensivists have increased in numbers, and many major institutions have attendings and fellowship programs. However, these books cross disciplines and should also be useful for intensivists, anesthesiologists, emergency physicians, nursing staff, and allied health care professionals in intensive care units and the emergency department. In the end the intent is to write a book that provides a sound reassuring basis to practice well, and that helps with understanding and appreciating the complexities of care of a patient with an acute neurologic condition.

1

Prognostication After Traumatic Brain Injury

Traumatic brain injury (TBI) affects millions of patients and places a burden on hospital care and rehabilitation. In younger individuals TBI is catastrophically costly.[14] Although TBI affects all ages, the largest database, created by the CRASH Trial Collaborators, reported more than 50% of TBIs occur in individuals older than 55 years of age. Most often, TBI involves males in a motor vehicle accident, with fatal outcome within the first two weeks in one out of five patients.[24] Frequently, TBI is associated with additional injury at the time of impact or appearing soon after as a result of severe hypoxemia and hypotension. As a result of military conflicts in Iraq and Afghanistan, TBI has been substantial and devastating for young troops.[31]

Any blow to the head may cause an obvious injury, but predicting the degree of recovery is complicated. A TBI may be categorized as closed with diffuse parenchymal lesions or extraparenchymal lesions such as subdural hematoma, closed with primary brainstem injury, or open due to projectiles—combinations can easily occur.

There has been advancement in prognostication due to the availability of two large cohorts (CRASH and IMPACT) of international patients.[19,20,24–26,30] Outcome in TBI is usually determined by the presence or absence of penetrating injury, pupil responses, unstable or refractory intracranial pressure (ICP), presence of associated multisystem injury, hypotension, and possibly socioeconomic status.[8,21,27,28,29,35]

It cannot be assumed that prognostication can be dissected into a simple set of clinical and radiological variables, but these rich data sets are as close to an estimation a physician can get. There are many unknowns in prognostication of TBI, and there is a significant part of actual patient care still poorly captured within large data set numbers. Some examples are early versus protracted recognition of major medical complications, early versus late treatment of shock, and early prophylaxis versus waiting for a complication to occur. Crucial questions remain: How can physicians make a considered judgment on future prognosis? Does a handful of predicting factors provide sufficient information in such a diverse spectrum of injuries? Is generalizing prognostic factors potentially of concern in this category of patients? What are the relevant clinical, radiological, and physiological factors that determine the likely course of a patient with severe TBI?

This chapter tries to answer these unavoidable questions and discusses the most important criteria and ways to prognosticate after TBI.

Principles

Traumatic brain injury results from a sequence of events and includes rapid changes in the cytoarchitecture of the traumatized neuron. Primary axotomy is the result of the mechanical insult, and secondary axotomy is a phase caused by pathological changes within the axon, resulting in major biochemical changes. The node of Ranvier is the weakest part of the axon, and that is where the disruption is most noticeable, resulting in swelling and eventually cytoskeletal disruption. Axonal transport is quickly impaired, and an inflammatory cascade starts, resulting in secondary neuronal injury.

Cerebral blood flow changes dramatically. There appears to be a multiphasic response of hypoperfusion in the first 24 hours followed by a hyperemic phase several days later—cerebral blood flow may decrease again due to cerebral vasospasm. Recently, it has also been found that in the case of a blast injury to the brain, cerebral vasospasm reducing cerebral blood flow occurs in up to 50% of patients and may last for weeks.[31] (more details are in volume *Handling Difficult Situations*) This simple summary indicates some basic crucial factors to note: degree of axonal injury, inflammatory markers, changes in cerebral perfusion, and appearance of swelling. Some fundamental knowledge is needed to adequately use models, biomarkers, and other clinical markers for prognostication. Here we discuss seven core principles.

First—Prognostication of acute TBI involves a full assessment of the severity of injury. TBI is rarely seen in isolation, and multiorgan injury may have to be taken into account. No decision can (or should) be made within the first days after presentation except in patients who are nearly fulfilling the clinical criteria of brain death. Despite pressures to deescalate care sufficient time of observation and aggressive initial management are necessary to assess the degree of injury. It is very common to be in a situation where clinical examination can be confounded by hypotension, laboratory abnormalities, or recent drug administration.

Second—Coma can result from different types of injuries. Traumatic brainstem injury may be the primary reason for coma in traumatic head injury and, due to significant force, is often combined with shear lesions at other locations. The outcome is largely determined by the size of the lesion. Nonpenetrating injury with primary brainstem injury has a much worse prognosis than other types of traumatic brain injury. These comatose patients have significant pontomesencephalic neuronal injury, and survival is not expected. The vast majority of comatose patients die without awakening, which is explained by a permanently injured reticular formation. Gunshot wounds to the head could result in prolonged coma due to diencephalic destruction, with a high mortality rate due to development of diffuse cerebral edema. Fixed pupils in a comatose patient with such a penetrating high velocity injury and without the presence of a potentially removable hematoma, indicate a poor outcome.

Third—It is essential to consider contributing confounding factors. Traumatic brain injury is commonly associated with alcohol or drug intoxication. However, it is more important to point out that several studies have found that when blood alcohol concentration was available, it did not appear to erroneously reduce the Glasgow Coma Scale in traumatic head injury patients.[2] More often, alcohol or drug intoxication is associated with increased injury severity.[38]

Physicians should recognize paroxysmal sympathetic hyperactivity (PSH) as an early but also a late phenomenon and confounder. PHS is frequently associated with worse neurologic outcome, with longer rehabilitation stays and more cognitive impairment, but treatment can be effective if PHS is recognized. Physicians who are unfamiliar with this complication may mistake these manifestations for a mere epiphenomenon of severe brain injury. They are rapid and episodic (i.e., paroxysmal) manifestations of excessive sympathetic activity. Patients become tachycardic, hypertensive (with increased pulse pressure), tachypneic, febrile, or diaphoretic; often they develop markedly increased muscle tone, which may result in posturing. Pupillary dilatation, piloerection, and skin flushing may also be seen. Paroxysmal sympathetic hyperactivity responds best to intermittent doses of morphine, scheduled doses of clonidine, and increasing doses of gabapentin.

Fourth—Treatment of traumatic brain injury is dependent on the aggressiveness of care. This is true with any model of prognostication in medicine, of course. A key moment in patient care is the decision to place a tracheostomy and a gastrostomy. This decision opens a pathway to aggressive and prolonged care and, much less likely, early withdrawal of support. In the United States, there might also be a strong financial benefit to placing a tracheostomy, as the procedure increases the diagnosis-related group reimbursement rate.[9]

Outcome after TBI is clearly determined by aggressive treatment of increased ICP, which could incorporate neurosurgical interventions including removal of contusions in patients with subdural hematomas, and other stabilizing measures.[7] Very few prognostic studies have specifically addressed ICP, and a recent comparative prospective trial on monitoring (yes or no) and effect of treatment—keeping ICP consistently below 20 mm Hg—found no effect on outcome.[5] Some studies have found that refractory ICP makes poor outcome six times more likely. Removal of a contusion or decompressive craniectomy may also be effective in selected patients and may change prognostic outlook.

Consistency of care is difficult to achieve in this heterogeneous population. Any data set that has a low incidence of neurosurgical procedures in severe traumatic head injury and a low percentage of tracheostomy might be biased toward early withdrawal of care after TBI. Protocol-driven or an individualized approach—with much more erratic management—may impact outcome.

Fifth—There may be biomarkers associated with structural damage. Ideally, a panel of biomarkers indicates the severity of brain injury. Point-of-care biomarker-based prognosticating tests are currently not available but could become useful if studies find high sensitivity and specificity.

Axonal biomarkers include neurofilament, usually degraded into fragments that can only be detected in cerebrospinal fluid (CSF). A bioassay of serum neurofilament-H is currently being developed. Another axonal biomarker is the microtubule-associated protein Tau and this may be useful in quantifying axonal injury. The utility of these axonal biomarkers is yet unclear, with some studies reporting poor predictive values.[33]

The major difficulties with using biomarkers are best illustrated with S100B, which is a marker of glial activation.[1,3] This calcium-binding protein is usually expressed in astrocytes but also in oligodendrocytes. However, serum S100B levels are already elevated in a third of the patients after minor head injury. S100B levels are also increased in patients who have sustained large bone fractures, abdominal injury, and other large extracranial injuries. S100B levels are very high in patients with gunshot wounds. Nonetheless, serum S100B does appear to be proportionally related to the severity of TBI and inversely proportional to the Glasgow outcome score.[32,36] Levels of S100B and neuron-specific enolase (NSE) have been found to be predictive in several studies.[15,17] In severe TBI, approximately half of the patients have elevated NSE (defined as more than 12 mcg/L) and increased S100B (defined as more than 0.1 mcg/L).[3]

Other possibly meaningful CSF biomarkers include glial fibrillary acidic protein (GFAP), ubiquitin C-terminal hydrolase-L1 (UCH-L1), and αII-spectrin breakdown product (SBDP). Preliminary studies suggest that these biomarkers maybe have predictive value beyond that derived from currently available clinical and neuroradiological data.[6] Neuroinflammation results in oxidative stress, and lipid peroxidation might also be a marker of neuronal injury. Inflammatory markers include C-reactive protein, matrix metalloproteinase-9, interleukin-6 (IL-6), tumor necrosis factor-alpha (TNF-α), and adhesion molecules. Earlier studies suggested that these markers may have prognosticating value, but unfortunately, multiple cutoff points have been proposed in predicting poor outcome.[34]

Sixth—Cerebral blood flow changes may be related to outcome after traumatic brain injury. Cerebral blood flow changes may be compartmentalized, with reduction in contused areas and focal hyperemia in the tissue approximating the contusion. Any of these global abnormalities—whether hypoperfusion or hyperemia—indicate a poor outcome. Reduced cerebral blood flow in the first week of injury is more often seen in patients with multiple cerebral contusions. Jugular venous oxygen desaturation has been associated with decreased cerebral blood flow and outcome was related to the number of desaturations. When cerebral metabolic rate of oxygen consumption is taken into account, the relationship with outcome becomes clearer. Conversely, high jugular venous oxygen desaturation could predict poor outcome if cerebral metabolic rate of oxygen consumption is decreased. High jugular venous oxygen desaturation could predict good outcome if cerebral blood flow is increased. (Cerebral oxygen delivery is cerebral blood flow multiplied by arterial oxygen concentration. Because arterial oxygen concentration and hemoglobin concentration are important factors, hypoxemia and anemia are relevant factors in the equation.)

Seventh—It is necessary to estimate the quality of life. After any TBI, it is important to assess how the patient performs and whether the patient is able to return to his prior occupation. After TBI, other issues play an important role. Outcome can be determined by illicit drug and alcohol consumption leading to leaving the hospital against medical advice.[9] Aggressiveness of rehabilitation may be a reflection of type of insurance. One study found that caucasians are significantly more likely than patients of other ethnicities to be discharged to rehabilitation centers rather than to home. These decisions may not necessarily be physician's bias but could also be a part of cultural beliefs, willingness of family members, and even lack of trust in the medical system.

All of these above components play an important role in assessing data on prognosis after TBI. It may all add up to a complex scenario that cannot be reduced to a few simple facts.

In Practice

No neurosurgeon, neurointensivist, or neurohospitalist will be able to see a sufficient number of patients to gain major experience in prognostication. Therefore, large databases are very helpful in assessing the chief factors. Both the IMPACT and CRASH studies have found several variables that consistently predict death or poor outcome. Guidelines for treatment may also be based on such cohorts.[4,5,13,14,23,28]

These databases have therefore supplanted multiple prognosticating studies that were limited by quality, small sample size, and management in high-income countries. Both IMPACT and CRASH studies found that strong predictors for outcome are age, motor response, pupil reactivity to light, and findings on an admission CT scan. Also entering secondary insults, including hypotension and hypoxemia, and laboratory variables, including blood glucose and hemoglobin, have improved the model.

However, although the databases provide excellent probabilistic estimates of outcome, originators of both databases argue against using them for prognostication. As expected, family members suddenly confronted with the patient's condition may have difficulty interpreting percentages. Furthermore, it has been known for years that statistically derived prediction models may reduce level of care rather than doing the opposite—result in an extra effort.[26] Missing data are also common concerns using these large databases and calculation models.

The CRASH study was international and was able to identify predictors depending on country of origin. The CRASH study included over 10,000 patients with 81% men and 75% from low- to middle-income countries. Nearly 20% died within the first two weeks, 24% died within 6 months, and 37% were dead or severely disabled at 6 months. Generally there was no association between age and mortality within the first 2 weeks before the age of 40, after which the relationship linearly increased. Coma was the strongest predictor of outcome in low- to middle-income countries, age was the strongest predictor in high-income countries, and pupil nonreactivity was the third-strongest predictor in both regions.

The investigators created a basic model of clinical features and a model incorporating CT results for predicting outcomes in two settings (low- to middle-income and high-income countries). Four predictors were included in the basic model: age, Glasgow Coma Scale (GCS), pupil reactivity, and the presence of major extracranial injury. Radiological characteristics on CT using the Marshall classification system (Table 1.1) were also strongly associated with outcome and included the presence of petechial hemorrhages, obliteration of the basal cisterns or third ventricle, subarachnoid hemorrhage, midline shift, and hematoma.

The International Mission for Prognosis and Analysis of Clinical Trials (IMPACT) in TBI study group grew as a collaborative venture and included investigators from Belgium, the Netherlands, the UK, and the United States. Over nearly a decade, data from more than 40,000 patients was gathered. IMPACT is also used for recommendations for design and analysis of clinical trials.

As the authors of both studies acknowledged, the external validity of the models may be limited to some degree because initially the patients came from a large clinical trial rather than from the general population, but this also allowed prospective and standardized collection of data, which increased the internal validity of the study. One of the limitations of the CRASH study is that the investigators in the initial trial did

Table 1.1 **Marshall CT Classification**

Class	Definition
Diffuse injury I	• No visible intracranial pathological changes seen on CT scan
Diffuse injury II	• Cisterns are present with midline shift of 0–5 mm and/or lesions present • No high- or mixed-density lesion >25 cm³ • May include bone fragments and foreign bodies*
Diffuse injury III (swelling)	• Cisterns compressed or absent with midline shift of 0–5 mm • No high- or mixed-density lesion >25 cm³
Diffuse injury IV (shift)	• Midline shift >5 mm • No high- or mixed-density lesion >25 cm³
Evacuated mass lesion	• Any lesion surgically evacuated
Nonevacuated mass lesion	• High- or mixed-density lesion >25 cm³; not surgically evacuated

*As may be the case in depressed skull fractures.

Source: With permission from reference 22.

Table 1.2 **Comparison of IMPACT and CRASH Prediction Models**

	Predicted Outcome	Core Model	CT Model	Laboratory Model
IMPACT	Mortality at 6 months or unfavorable outcome at 6 months	Age, motor score, pupil reactivity	Core model plus: hypoxia, hypotension, CT classification, traumatic subarachnoid hemorrhage on CT, epidural mass on CT	Core model plus: glucose and hemoglobin concentrations
CRASH	Mortality at 14 days or unfavorable outcome at 6 months	Age, GCS score, pupil reactivity, major extracranial injury	Core model plus: petechial hemorrhages, obliteration of the third ventricle or basal cisterns, subarachnoid bleeding, midline shift, nonevacuated hematoma	

CRASH = Corticosteroid Randomization After Significant Head Injury. GCS = Glasgow coma scale. IMPACT = International Mission for Prognosis and Clinical Trial design in TBI. TBI = traumatic brain injury.

Source: With permission from reference 18.

not report the circumstances of death. Approximately 20% of the patients died within the first two weeks. Whether the limitation of aggressive medical or surgical care—or withdrawal of life-sustaining treatments in patients—was associated with the presence of the prognostic variables later studied (older age, lower GCS, and nonreactive pupils, major extracranial injury, among other factors) is not known. The major components of both models are shown in Table 1.2, and the calculators available online (www.crash.lshtm.ac.uk and www.tbi-impact.org) are shown in Figure 1.1.

A degree of uncertainty in prognostication after TBI is unavoidable, but the results of this study have greatly assisted clinicians in making therapeutic decisions and counseling patients and their relatives. One example illustrates how using these calculators in clinical practice can be tricky (something the investigators freely acknowledge): An 18-year-old comatose patient in the United States with TBI and extensor posturing, CT Marshall grade III (diffuse swelling), and no other major abnormalities will have a 45% likelihood of death at 14 days and 76% poor outcome at 6 months based on CRASH and 39% mortality at 6 months and 67% unfavorable outcome based on IMPACT. These mortality figures—the glass half full or half empty argument—will have limited use.

The aggressiveness of neurosurgical intervention impacts outcome. Neurosurgical decompression of extraaxial subdural hematoma may result in seizures and prolonged stupor, a phenomenon that has not been clearly understood.

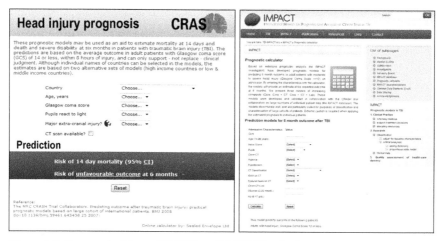

Figure 1.1 Screen shot from CRASH and IMPACT calculators.

Despite adequate removal of the subdural hematoma, patients may take weeks to improve—some need close monitoring for seizures.

Decompressive craniectomy as a treatment for intractable increased ICP has been studied and resulted in a 6-month postoperative mortality rate around 30%.[10] This option also led to a reasonably good quality of life, but did not impact outcome in a large clinical trial (DECRA). The DECRA trial randomized 155 adults and found no improvement after decompressive craniectomy. The results of this trial are debated, and the design has been criticized for group imbalance and intervention at relatively low ICPs. Marked differences of pupil reactivity between the surgical and medically treated group might have impacted outcome.[37] The value of decompressive craniectomy on outcome after TBI therefore remains unclear, and it should remain reserved for patients who have refractory intracranial hypertension despite aggressive measures. A more recent study still placed mortality at more than 25% after craniectomy for TBI.[11]

In summary, a multimodal approach to prognostication using multiple components has a better predictive power than a single variable alone. Prognostication, for example, on the basis of neuroimaging, whether this represents CT or MRI scan, may lead to misjudgments and should be avoided. Every practitioner in this field knows that patients with large contusions, early brain edema, and initial poor neurological condition may still make a substantial improvement in a matter of months after TBI. However, if all of the factors can be evaluated reliably, some estimate is very helpful in determining long-term care and treatment of complications. Whether it provides realistic information for family members remains uncertain.

It is also useful to briefly revisit the rehabilitation trajectory. Patients who become severely disabled after severe TBI may be able to return to work in sheltered workplaces, usually with responsibilities far inferior to those before the injury. Visual difficulties due to cranial nerve involvement, central causes of vertigo, and more-difficult-to-measure panic and fear attacks resembling acute stress reaction are common and may limit ability to rejoin the workforce. Cognitive dysfunction is substantial after TBI and is the cause of decreased functional independence. The same applies for aggressive agitation common in 70% of patients admitted to rehabilitation centers. Only a relative minority are cared for in nursing homes. Depression and apathy, which may occur in combination, may respond to dopaminergic medication such as selegiline, bromocriptine, and amantadine. Many rehabilitation physicians prescribe psychostimulants. Post-traumatic stress disorder with major emotional and behavior abnormalities may occur, with or without objective findings of brain injury and cognitive rehabilitation in combat veterans is currently an active field of research within the Department of Veterans Affairs.

Here are some other facts. Improvement in traumatic head injury in hospitalized patients is different from that in patients in specialized rehabilitation centers. Length of coma is an unreliable predictor, because sedation may have been used to control agitation or ICP or mechanical ventilation. Once the patient awakens, simple motor skills improve over time. Following a craniotomy, patients may have major mood disturbances, headache, and long-standing fatigue. They may develop a full-blown trephine syndrome with a delayed contralateral hemiparesis, improving with cranioplasty Paradoxical herniation with progressive stupor may occur when a lumbar puncture is done to exclude meningitis. A negative pressure gradient exists between the cranial and spinal compartment, and CSF removal exacerbates that gradient. Mannitol can worsen the condition. Treatment is opposite that for "herniation". Trendelenburg positioning and blood patching of the lumbar puncture site are needed. Cranioplasty repair reverses these complications.

So how do patients fare after a severe TBI, and what can we (and families) expect? It only takes a minute on the Web to find stories of "miracle" patients who made an "unexpected" recovery or awoke from a supposedly "vegetative state" after physicians had given up on them. What is the reality? Persistent vegetative state (PVS) mostly occurs in polytraumatized critically ill patients but remains uncommon and most patients are in a minimally conscious state (MCS). PVS becomes clear 1 month after TBI when patients open their eyes and develop sleep-wake cycles. It may take one full year to confidently consider it permanent. Recovery from a prolonged PVS to a more responsive minimally conscious state has been documented in only a few cases.

By the Way

- The heterogeneity of TBI limits prognostication
- Sports related severe TBI ends sports careers
- Prognostication in young individuals remains unreliable
- MRI has remained unreliable as an absolute predictor of poor outcome
- Persistent vegetative state is rare after TBI
- Rehabilitation options may be limited in severe TBI

Prognostication of Traumatic Brain Injury by the Numbers

- ~50% of comatose patients with TBI improve significantly in 6 months
- ~25% of patients with severe TBI will have a major depression
- ~20% of patients with penetrating TBI will develop epilepsy
- ~10% of comatose patients with TBI transition to MCS
- ~5% of comatose patients with TBI progress to brain death
- ~5% of comatose patients with TBI transition to PVS after 12 months

---

Putting It All Together

- Outcome after TBI can be assessed with reasonable certainty, but caveats remain
- Outcome after TBI requires a complex approach to prognostication using multiple components
- The impact of ICP monitoring on outcome after TBI remains unclear
- The impact of decompressive craniectomy on outcome after TBI remains unclear

References

1. Anderson RE, Hansson LO, Nilsson O, Dijlai-Merzoug R, Settergren G. High serum S100B levels for trauma patients without head injuries. *Neurosurgery* 2001;48:1255–1258.
2. Berry C, Salim A, Alban R, et al. Serum ethanol levels in patients with moderate to severe traumatic brain injury influence outcomes: a surprising finding. *Am Surg* 2010;76:1067–1070.
3. Bloomfield SM, McKinney J, Smith L, Brisman J. Reliability of S100B in predicting severity of central nervous system injury. *Neurocrit Care* 2007;6:121–138.
4. Brain Trauma Foundation; American Association of Neurological Surgeons; Congress of Neurological Surgeons. Guidelines for the management of severe traumatic brain injury. *J Neurotrauma* 2007;24:S1–S106.
5. Chesnut RM, Temkin N, Carney N, et al. A trial of intracranial-pressure monitoring in traumatic brain injury. *N Engl J Med* 2012;367:2471–2481.

6. Czeiter E, Mondello S, Kovacs N, et al. Brain injury biomarkers may improve the predictive power of the IMPACT outcome calculator. *J Neurotrauma* 2012;29:1770–1778.

7. Danish SF, Barone D, Lega BC, Stein SC. Quality of life after hemicraniectomy for traumatic brain injury in adults: a review of the literature. *Neurosurg Focus* 2009;26:E2.

8. De Silva MJ, Roberts I, Perel P, et al. Patient outcome after traumatic brain injury in high-, middle- and low-income countries: analysis of data on 8927 patients in 46 countries. *Int J Epidemiol* 2009;38:452–458.

9. Heffernan DS, Vera RM, Monaghan SF, et al. Impact of socioethnic factors on outcomes following traumatic brain injury. *J Trauma* 2011;70:527–534.

10. Ho KM, Honeybul S, Lind CR, Gillett GR, Litton E. Cost-effectiveness of decompressive craniectomy as a lifesaving rescue procedure for patients with severe traumatic brain injury. *J Trauma* 2011;71:1637–1644.

11. Huang YH, Lee TC, Lee TH, Liao CC, Sheehan J, Kwan AL. Thirty-day mortality in traumatically brain-injured patients undergoing decompressive craniectomy. *J Neurosurg* 2013;118:1329–1335.

12. Hukkelhoven CW, Steyerberg EW, Habbema JD, et al. Predicting outcome after traumatic brain injury: development and validation of a prognostic score based on admission characteristics. *J Neurotrauma* 2005;22:1025–1039.

13. Hyam JA, Welch CA, Harrison DA, Menon DK. Case mix, outcomes and comparison of risk prediction models for admissions to adult, general and specialist critical care units for head injury: a secondary analysis of the ICNARC Case Mix Programme Database. *Crit Care* 2006;10 Suppl 2:S2.

14. Hyder AA, Wunderlich CA, Puvanachandra P, Gururaj G, Kobusingye OC. The impact of traumatic brain injuries: a global perspective. *NeuroRehabilitation* 2007;22:341–353.

15. Kochanek PM, Berger RP, Bayir H, et al. Biomarkers of primary and evolving damage in traumatic and ischemic brain injury: diagnosis, prognosis, probing mechanisms, and therapeutic decision making. *Curr Opin Crit Care* 2008;14:135–141.

16. Leitgeb J, Mauritz W, Brazinova A, et al. Effects of gender on outcomes after traumatic brain injury. *J Trauma* 2011;71:1620–1626.

17. Li J, Li XY, Feng DF, Pan DC. Biomarkers associated with diffuse traumatic axonal injury: exploring pathogenesis, early diagnosis, and prognosis. *J Trauma* 2010;69: 1610–1618.

18. Lingsma HF, Roozenbeek B, Steyerberg EW, Murray GD, Maas AI. Early prognosis in traumatic brain injury: from prophecies to predictions. *Lancet Neurol* 2010;9:543–554.

19. Maas AI, Marmarou A, Murray GD, Teasdale SG, Steyerberg EW. Prognosis and clinical trial design in traumatic brain injury: the IMPACT study. *J Neurotrauma* 2007;24:232–238.

20. Maas AI, Roozenbeek B, Manley GT. Clinical trials in traumatic brain injury: past experience and current developments. *Neurotherapeutics* 2010;7:115–126.

21. Marmarou A, Anderson RL, Ward JD, et al. Impact of ICP instability and hypotension on outcome in patients with severe head trauma. *J Neurosurg* 1991;75:s59–s66.

22. Marshall LF, Bowers S, Klauber MR, et al. A new classification of head injury based on computerised tomography. *J Neurosurg* 1991;75:1:S14–S20.

23. Menon DK, Zahed C. Prediction of outcome in severe traumatic brain injury. *Curr Opin Crit Care* 2009;15:437–441.

24. MRC CRASH Trial Collaborators, Perel P, Arango M, et al. Predicting outcome after traumatic brain injury: practical prognostic models based on large cohort of international patients. *BMJ* 2008;336:425–429.

25. Murray GD, Butcher I, McHugh GS, et al. Multivariable prognostic analysis in traumatic brain injury: results from the IMPACT study. *J Neurotrauma* 2007;24:329–337.

26. Murray LS, Teasdale GM, Murray GD, et al. Does prediction of outcome alter patient management? *Lancet* 1993;341:1487–1491.

27. Ono J, Yamaura A, Kubota M, Okimura Y, Isobe K. Outcome prediction in severe head injury: analyses of clinical prognostic factors. *J Clin Neurosci* 2001;8:120–123.

28. Patel HC, Bouamra O, Woodford M, et al. Trends in head injury outcome from 1989 to 2003 and the effect of neurosurgical care: an observational study. *Lancet* 2005;366:1538–1544.

29. Perel P, Edwards P, Wentz R, Roberts I. Systematic review of prognostic models in traumatic brain injury. *BMC Med Inform Decis Mak* 2006;6:38.

30. Roozenbeek B, Chiu YL, Lingsma HF, et al. Predicting 14-day mortality after severe traumatic brain injury: application of the IMPACT models in the Brain Trauma Foundation TBI-trac(®) New York State Database. *J Neurotrauma* 2012;29:1306–1312.

31. Rosenfeld JV, McFarlane AC, Bragge P, Armonda RA, Grimes JB, Ling GS. Blast-related traumatic brain injury. *Lancet Neurol* 2013;12:882–893.

32. Schültke E, Sadanand V, Kelly ME, Griebel RW, Juurlink BH. Can admission S-100beta predict the extent of brain damage in head trauma patients? *Can J Neurol Sci* 2009;36:612–616.

33. Teunissen CE, Dijkstra C, Polman C. Biological markers in CSF and blood for axonal degeneration in multiple sclerosis. *Lancet Neurol* 2005;4:32–41.

34. Topolovec-Vranic J, Pollmann-Mudryj MA, Ouchterlony D, et al. The value of serum biomarkers in prediction models of outcome after mild traumatic brain injury. *J Trauma* 2011;71:S478–S486.

35. Treggiari MM, Schutz N, Yanez ND, Romand JA. Role of intracranial pressure values and patterns in predicting outcome in traumatic brain injury: a systematic review. *Neurocrit Care* 2007;6:104–112.

36. Vos PE, Lamers KJ, Hendriks JC, et al. Glial and neuronal proteins in serum predict outcome after severe traumatic brain injury. *Neurology* 2004;62:1303–1310.

37. Walcott BP, Kahle KT, Simard JM. The DECRA trial and decompressive craniectomy in diffuse traumatic brain injury: is decompression really ineffective? *World Neurosurg* 2013;79:80–81.

38. West SL. Substance use among persons with traumatic brain injury: a review. *NeuroRehabilitation* 2011;29:1–8.

2

Prognostication After Ischemic
or Hemorrhagic Stroke

The category "stroke" includes several major cerebrovascular disorders, which are subdivided into clinical syndromes. Mainly these syndromes are due to large or small (penetrating) artery occlusions, intracerebral hemorrhage, and subarachnoid hemorrhage. Less common are cerebral venous occlusions. There is a reasonably good understanding of the pathophysiology in each of these disorders, and one can imagine that detailed neuroimaging and multicenter experience with large numbers of patients with an acute stroke over the years should have provided indisputable data on outcome—alas, the current situation is quite the opposite.

If all strokes and medical comorbidities are taken together and a focal neurologic deficit is assessed by nonspecialists, outcome apparently can be predicted.[36] Oversimplification of a complex disease process with differing etiologies, however, may trigger a failure to recognize time-limited treatment options in patients with a presumed poor outcome.[9] Very few, if any, studies have empirically tested the accuracy of neurologists, neurosurgeons, or emergency physicians in predicting outcome in stroke; none have focused on what elements physicians use to come to such a prediction.[34]

Most important in this regard for neurologists is to have a good sense of whether the patient has even a chance of survival in a functional state. Causes of early mortality are known, and few can be prevented. Knowing prognosis in certain types of stroke could also lead to finding interventions that could improve prognosis. So, if absent corneal reflexes from brainstem compression portend a poor prognosis in cerebellar hematoma, then—potentially—early removal of the hematoma may change the clinical course.

The inevitable heterogeneity of hemorrhagic and ischemic stroke and the different prior comorbid states would seem to preclude robust prognostication.[5,6] Many factors play a role in determining prognosis, and in only some patients is it determined almost immediately at onset. The outcome of a stroke in a patient with multiple prior cardiac interventions, advanced cancer, or even a serious metabolic syndrome might be notably different from the outcome of a stroke in a "previously healthy" elderly patient. Equally important is the question of whether interventions matter. The way acute presentations are approached by the physician who sees the patient first may impact the outcome, particularly if the very first decisions that are made are inefficient or inappropriate. A good example is failure to immediately reverse anticoagulation with rapidly acting agents in a patient with a cerebral hemorrhage.[41] In the last 10 years or so, outcome in major ischemic stroke has become fully dependent on a multidisciplinary assessment and a readily available neurointerventionalist team but this pathway should be known.

Once the patient survives and support is given to allow recovery, the availability of comprehensive multispecialty rehabilitation becomes important. We all have seen continuous improvement in a patient months after discharge.

How can we best assess morbidity in stroke, and what is the pattern of improvement if there is any? Are there critical junctures where we can say with sufficient confidence that the observed deficit is permanent? How can physicians best grade outcome in stroke and interpret the patient's well-being? This chapter describes in more detail the practice of prognostication and points out the clinical metrics used in major stroke syndromes.

Principles

Scales are best judged by practicality, communicability, and reproducibility. A stroke often leaves patients with a new reality and much different quality of life. None of the scales takes into account the level of care or where the patient is managed (i.e., general ward, stroke unit, general medical intensive care unit, or neurosciences intensive care unit). There are three major principles: what scale to use, what scale to use in what disorder, and when to assess patients.

Measuring outcome in stroke has certainly improved with numerous stroke trials.[17,20,28,50] Although multiple scores and scales have been published, the modified Rankin scale (mRs; Table 2.1) has been universally adopted and dichotomized to show poor versus good or reasonably good outcome. Training in use of the mRs can be found online (www.rankinscale.org). A 90-day mRs has been used in

Table 2.1 **The Modified Rankin Scale (mRS)**

0	No symptoms.
1	No significant disability. Able to carry out all usual activities, despite some symptoms.
2	Slight disability. Able to look after own affairs without assistance, but unable to carry out all previous activities.
3	Moderate disability. Requires some help, but able to walk unassisted.
4	Moderately severe disability. Unable to attend to own bodily needs without assistance, and unable to walk unassisted.
5	Severe disability. Requires constant nursing care and attention, bedridden, incontinent.
6	Dead.

virtually all acute stroke trials and is established as a useful metric. The mRs measures the degree of disability and dependency in daily activities.[28] It is scored on an ordinal scale from 0 to 6. In each study, it is important to see whether the Rankin scale is used appropriately and what is understood by a poor or good outcome. The mRs has been divided into a Rankin scale of 0–2 and >2, 0–3 and >3, and 0–4 and >4.[55] The scale, however, is not specific to stroke. Other outcome measures are the National Institutes of Health Stroke Scale (NIHSS), the Barthel index,[30] and the Glasgow Outcome Score. The Euro-Qol visual analogue scale (from 0 to 100) is a self-rating health quality-of-life rating.[49] Another widely used metric is the functional independence measure, which is based on how much assistance is needed to perform important activities of daily living. These are eating, grooming, bathing, sphincter control, mobility, locomotion, communication, and social cognition. The instrument is graded on a 7-point ordinal scale (Table 2.2).[31] The scale is useful for tabulation, but it remains difficult to find the most clinically relevant change in score, and it may also be dependent on baseline score. The scores range from 18 to 126. One study found changes in scores had to be large in order to represent notable improvement: in total FIM score, 22 points; in the motor part of the FIM score, 17 points; in the cognitive part of the FIM score, 3 points.[7] Prognostic algorithm models are not available in ischemic stroke (except in anoxic-ischemic injury to the brain; Chapter 3). The NIHSS does assess severity, and higher scores (>16) have—in older studies before endovascular intervention—been linked to higher likelihood of mortality.

Table 2.2 **Functional Independence Measure (FIM) Rating Scale**

FIM Rating	Definition
1	Maximum dependence—Patient performs less than 25% of the task
2	Patient can perform 25%–49% of the task, the remaining 50%–75% dependent on the caregiver or assistive device
3	Patient can perform 50%–74% of the task, the remaining 25%–50% being performed by the caregiver or device
4	Patient can perform ≥75% of the task and requires ≤25% from the caregiver
5	Supervision—Patient requires verbal cuing or set-up to perform the task; caregiver needs to be on "stand-by" or "contact guard" assist
6	Modified independent—Patient can perform with assistive devices, or with increased time; no assistance required from the caregiver
7	Complete independence

Dimensions assessed include: Eating; Grooming; Bathing; Upper body dressing; Lower body dressing; Toileting; Bladder management; Bowel management; Bed to chair transfer; Toilet transfer; Shower transfer; Locomotion (ambulatory or wheelchair level); Stairs; Cognitive comprehension; Expression; Social interaction; Problem solving; Memory.

Prognostic scales have been developed for cerebral hemorrhage and many are highly predictive of 30-day mortality.[37] Two such scores are the intracerebral hemorrhage (ICH) and FUNC scores,[24,47] which reflect clinical findings and initial neuroimaging results. None of the scales can avoid the pitfall that presumption of poor outcome may have impacted the level of care. In other words, large-volume hemorrhages in the elderly may not receive the aggressive approach used in small hemorrhages in young patients. Initial stroke severity is—expectedly—a predictor of poor outcome. Other scales have included intraventricular hemorrhage temperature, pulse pressure, glucose level, and dialysis dependency, among other factors. Other scales have been modifications of each other. Some scales in cerebral hemorrhage include the Glasgow Coma Scale total score, volume of intracranial hemorrhage above or below tentorium, location of the hemorrhage, age, and more recently, presence of comorbidities. Many of the scales do not have sufficient external validation or are not as accurate in determining mortality. The scales in cerebral hemorrhage are unreliable in patients with cerebral hemorrhage associated with a ruptured aneurysm or hemorrhage associated with arteriovenous malformation (AVM).

One of the most important principles in determining outcome after a major stroke is distinguishing comatose patients from patients who are not comatose and determining whether there is already an associated brainstem injury. For example, a large lobar hematoma resulting in a loss of upper brainstem reflexes (such as pupil and corneal reflexes) markedly decreases the chance of a satisfactory outcome even after immediate neurosurgical intervention. Placement of a ventriculostomy in acute obstructive hydrocephalus in cerebral hemorrhage is an important determinant of outcome. Many studies have found that acute hydrocephalus in cerebral hemorrhage leads to poor outcome with or without ventriculostomy placement. These clinical findings trump all other variables used to prognosticate.

A second principle is that the timing of assessment for outcome is important. Most physicians will refrain from any categorical statements early after presentation, and assessment of the patient for prognostic purposes should be after all resuscitative measures have been tried. For example, most studies in subarachnoid hemorrhage use the Hunt and Hess and WFNS scale, and timing of assessment greatly affects prognostication. A poor WFNS after resuscitation has a better prognostic value than when assessed before "stabilization" of the patient.[15] This may include even a simple measure such as recognizing and treating seizures, aspiration, or a coexisting major infection.

In Practice

Many patients are affected greatly by stroke, and their lives change abruptly. Mobility and adequate communication remain important factors in determining outcome after a stroke. Poor outcome may not be that "poor" for some family members, but may be absolutely devastating for others. Patients' families should be informed that poor outcomes may necessitate nursing home placement due to full dependence on nursing care. The situation becomes difficult when less disabled patients, who may not require 24-hour nursing care, are discharged to the community without adequate support or follow-up.

GENERAL OBSERVATIONS DURING RECOVERY

Recovery potential and rehabilitation opportunities are obviously important factors but often it is not possible to say that improvement will occur with certainty. Recovery from major disabling symptoms such as aphasia, hemiplegia, or ophthalmoplegia—once ischemic stroke is established and cerebral hemorrhage is stable—is variable, as expected, and likely nonlinear. Aphasia after stroke may improve up to 6 months after stroke, after which it may reach a plateau. Semantics and syntax may improve significantly up to 6 weeks; phonology and token test (measuring severity of aphasia) may improve up to 3 months. In patients with global aphasia, speech output may improve, but verbal communication lags significantly behind.[3,12] To a certain degree, and depending on the severity of aphasia, outcome may be influenced by speech therapy.

Recovery from hemiplegia may take much longer, with many patients paretic and without function 6 months after the event.[48] Arm function recovery is much less expected than leg function recovery.[11,27] Voluntary finger extensions and shoulder abduction within a week of stroke predicts further recovery.[35] If both movements are absent, only 1 in 10 recover any (mostly nonfunctional) dexterity.[35] Increasing tone in one or both legs will allow a patient to stand, but walking is very difficult to predict at the outset, although there is reason for optimism if standing with little assistance (i.e., a supporting arm) can be achieved.

Neglect after stroke may improve, but approximately one-third of patients will have clear signs of neglect a full year after the stroke, which will interfere with rehabilitation of a paretic limb and transfers.[43,26] Dysphagia is also markedly worse in patients with persistent neglect, with dribbling and potential for choking and aspiration.[1]

Whether functional MRI or transcranial magnetic stimulation can be used to predict recovery is not yet known, but early results are promising. Repeated transcranial magnetic stimulation may increase corticomotor activity and, ideally, improve functional reorganization and neural plasticity.

Predictors for functional outcome after ischemic and hemorrhagic stroke are age, prior stroke, urinary incontinence, abnormal consciousness and disorientation at onset, sitting balance, and degree of social support. This information is broad, and it is best to further discuss outcome by type of stroke.

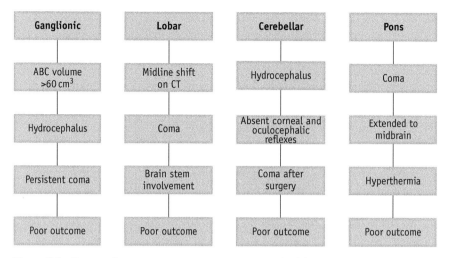

Figure 2.1   Factors determining poor outcome in cerebral hemorrhage.

INTRACEREBRAL HEMORRHAGE

Some general observations have emerged, and there has been an agreement that patient age greater than 70 years, a decreased level of consciousness after the ictus, severe limb hemiparesis, a large-clot hemorrhage (defined as more than 60 cm³ by ABC method (largest diameter [A], largest diameter 90° to A on same slice [B], and approximate number of 10 mm slices on which hematoma is seen [C]; A, B, C are multiplied and divided by 2), hematoma growth[10], presence of intraventricular blood (more than 20 cm³), presence of midline structure shift of more than 1 cm, and acute hydrocephalus in a ganglionic hemorrhage are all strong indicators of poor outcome[39,40] (Figure 2.1).

Neurosurgical intervention may change outcome. However, two major clinical trials (STICH I–STICH II) have not shown improved outcome after surgical intervention in stable patients with ICH.[32,33] The need for clot evacuation is often first determined by the site of the lesion. Deep ganglionic hemorrhages in the thalamus and putamen often extend to the ventricular system and cause acute hydrocephalus filled with clot. Mortality increases significantly without placement of ventriculostomy, but outcome is rarely improved with a ventriculostomy. The practice of ventriculostomy placement with subsequent infusion of tissue plasminogen activator (tPA) in patients with acutely dilated hemoventricles may clear CT scans (from clot resolution or preventing a drain from clotting off), but there is no convincing evidence that outcome is affected. Hemorrhages into the cerebellum need to be removed immediately, particularly if there is brainstem compression or extension to the vermis, and certainly if the patient is clinically deteriorating—even slightly so. Outcome is clearly linked to whether a suboccipital decompressive craniotomy is performed or whether a ventriculostomy is placed at the same time. Without this intervention, outcome is very poor. Neurosurgeons may be reluctant to proceed in elderly patients, and that in itself may link age to outcome.

Moreover, it is important to determine whether there is a spontaneous hemorrhage or a hemorrhage from an underlying vascular lesion. Usually, AVMs will present with hemorrhage (as opposed to headaches or seizures) at rates of 32% to 82% in reported large series.[2] Hemorrhage from an AVM obviously has a different outcome than a spontaneous intracranial hemorrhage because rehemorrhage changes patient prognosis significantly. Mortality doubles from 3% to 6% after recurrent hemorrhages.[2,37] A cerebral angiogram should be done urgently to determine the risk of rehemorrhage. Early rebleeding (within days to weeks of rupture) is uncommon but may be seen in patients with an AVM and a large associated varix.

The long-term risk of a rehemorrhage of an AVM increases in the first year and then may reduce itself to approximately 2% per year for up to 20 years. This compares with the lifetime risk of hemorrhage in a patient with an unruptured AVM which is 105 minus patient age in years in percentage. Thus, a 25-year-old patient with AVM will have a lifetime risk of hemorrhage of 105 − 25 = 80%.[8]

Acute neurosurgical removal of a ruptured AVM is likely warranted. Some centers have noted significant improvement with an early intervention, while others noted significant comorbidity after surgery. Most experts feel that aggressive and early management of a recent ruptured AVM often results in a favorable outcome with improved and accelerated rehabilitation.[2,37]

Outcome in cerebral hemorrhage is also determined by treatment of the complications of intracranial hemorrhage, including how quickly anticoagulation was reversed, use of osmotic diuretics with development of perihematomal edema,[38] and treatment of seizures. A few studies have noted that seizures have been associated with poor outcome.[9,14,25,29,38,51,59]

More recently, medical complications such as hyperglycemia have been identified as markers of poor prognosis.[4] Aggressive treatment of hyperglycemia has not been proven to impact outcome, although most institutions will use an insulin sliding scale to correct glucose to more normal values. Pulmonary status is an important determinant in any acute brain injury. Chronic pulmonary disease is more common in patients with a recent stroke, which predisposes them to pulmonary complications.[18] Outcome is not impacted by the need of a tracheostomy, and its placement allows quicker weaning from the ventilator. Whether any major pulmonary complication, such as aspiration, predicts outcome is not yet established, but the development of aspiration, pulmonary infection, pleural effusions, and atelectasis all may jeopardize patient's ability to recover.[4,23,39,42] One major medical complication is pulmonary embolus with a 1% incidence within three months after an intracranial hemorrhage. The risk is higher in patients not treated with subcutaneous heparin (usually started several days after onset). There is about 40% risk of deep venous thrombosis (dependent on use of regular surveillance with ultrasound). There is also approximately 10%–20% risk of a gastrointestinal bleed when unprotected by antacids. Each of these complications could reduce survival.

How does this bear on clinical practice? First, one should avoid unnecessary delay in treatment by acknowledging that there is a window of tissue vulnerability and by quickly acting on it. Second, one should follow the simple principles of explaining cause of coma in stroke. Becoming comatose after a stroke is an ominous sign and usually an indication of major tissue destruction. Most clinical signs pertain to primary or secondary (i.e., displacement from hemispheric or cerebellar lesion) brainstem injury. Failure to consider a neurosurgical intervention may lead to a much worse outcome if the hemorrhage is hemispheric lobar, cerebellar, or intraventricular.[32]

ANEURYSMAL SUBARACHNOID HEMORRHAGE

The clinical outcome in subarachnoid hemorrhages is very difficult to predict during hospital care. Still, many patients (1 out of 10) do reach the hospital in a moribund state and cannot be helped.[21] The remaining patients await a cerebral angiogram that shows the aneurysm and its configuration and size determines management. In the first weeks, outcome in aneurysmal subarachnoid hemorrhage is largely determined by deterioration from rebleeding, acute hydrocephalus, and delayed cerebral ischemia, but clipping may cause postoperative morbidity; coiling may need retreatment; flow diversion (pipeline) may cause thrombotic complications. These complications are associated with significant residual neurologic deficit and could change the outlook. Nevertheless, presentation in a poor-grade (or more simply defined as comatose) does not necessarily imply a poor outcome, and 1 out of 5 patients may still have a good outcome without cognitive defects. Approximately 20% of the patients after subarachnoid hemorrhage will remain markedly impaired (rated as an mRs score of 4 to 5). Moreover, in patients with aneurysmal subarachnoid hemorrhage it is also well known that outcome and life expectancy may be reduced due to other vascular events.[44,45,46,56]

Long-term outcome may change, and of patients who are discharged to a nursing home significantly disabled, one in three improves and recovers independent functioning within the first two years after admission.[16,17] Fifty percent of aneurysmal subarachnoid hemorrhage survivors who regain functional independence note some cognitive impairment, including dissatisfaction with their quality of life.

Generally, half of the patients have memory deficits that will persist beyond a year after aneurysmal subarachnoid hemorrhage.[17] In the second year after aneurysmal subarachnoid hemorrhage, a substantial number of the patients may face depression or anxiety. All of these complications may impact quality of life, ability to resume responsibilities, and return to work with major responsibilities.

The risk of a recurrent aneurysmal subarachnoid hemorrhage after coil treatment for the first one is low—approximately 3% in the first 10 years—and it could be lower if major risk factors such as smoking and hypertension are controlled. Aneurysm recurrence is associated with size of the aneurysm, neck width, suboptimal angiographic occlusion, and length of follow-up. Only 3% of aneurysm with narrow necks will need to be retreated. Unstable remnants appear to have a rebleed rate of 8%, which is higher than patients who have stable findings on follow-up imaging (<0.5%). Rebleeding rate within 30 days of endovascular treatment is approximately 1% and also related to the extent of remnant aneurysm.[13] Additional unruptured aneurysms that are found in a patient with aneurysmal subarachnoid hemorrhage will need to be followed up, but in the first years enlargement occurs in less than 5% of patients. At the 10-year follow-up mark, one in four aneurysms enlarge, but rarely notably.[57]

ISCHEMIC STROKES

Prognosticators for outcome of ischemic stroke are different for a stroke in the anterior cerebral circulation (carotid or middle cerebral artery) or a stroke in the posterior circulation (vertebral or basilar artery). Most outcome studies have concentrated on hemispheric (anterior circulation) ischemic stroke and whether cerebral edema emerges. The presence of hyperglycemia, multiple territorial strokes, early brain swelling within 24 hours, and failure to proceed with craniectomy all are factors associated with poor outcome[52] (Figure 2.2).

In a hemispheric stroke (i.e., middle cerebral artery), outcome can be poor or very unsatisfactory with no decompressive craniectomy or when it is performed

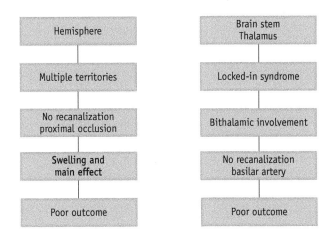

Figure 2.2 Factors determining poor outcome in ischemic stroke.

in the elderly (there is a continuum with much lesser benefit after the age of 60–70). Early versus late decompressive craniectomy also impacts outcome, with the preponderance of evidence suggesting that early decompression before the patient develops clinical signs of deterioration is more beneficial.[19,22,33,52,53,58] Adjunctive measures such as therapeutic hypothermia may not improve outcome. Full supportive and resuscitative measures, use of hypertonic saline (to avoid kidney injury with mannitol), and aggressive fever control may all impact outcome both in patients who were treated with decompressive craniectomy and in those who were not. If the physician and family decide against hemicraniectomy and then decide to transfer the patient with a hemispheric stroke outside a high level of care, outcome most definitively will be negatively affected.

Infarcts in the posterior circulation are mostly benign, and many brainstem strokes (with their many variants) have a good functional outcome. Cerebellar infarct, infarcts in the thalami (particularly when bilateral), or infarct in the occipital lobe can be quite disabling, impairing stance and motility, vision, and speech. An embolus in the posterior circulation in the basilar artery that causes coma or locked-in syndrome is associated with high mortality and often little recovery. In general, long-term care of patients with massive pontine infarcts cannot be expected to lead to a good functional outcome. Bilateral infarcts of the posterior cerebral artery can also be quite disabling, causing a Balint syndrome (inability to perceive the entire visual field as a whole) or cortical blindness with very protracted and often only moderate recovery.

By the Way

- Care of a stroke patient at home is life changing
- Depression may remain years after a stroke
- Dantrolene is helpful for hypertonic spasms
- Poststroke patients remain very susceptible to dehydration
- Obesity develops in many immobilized patients

Stroke Outcome By the Numbers

- ~90% of patients with a global aphasia improve in 1 month
- ~70% of patients cannot effectively swallow after a stroke
- ~50% of patients after a major stroke have persistent incontinence
- ~30% of patients have marked intellectual decline after a stroke
- ~30% of patients with a nondominant stroke have neglect after 6 months
- ~20% of patients after a stroke develop painful shoulder in hemiparetic arm

Putting It All Together

- Coma and involvement of the brainstem (absence of some or all cranial nerve reflexes) determines outcome in cerebral hemorrhage
- Hemispheric stroke with swelling (cerebellar or hemispheric) is associated with a poor outcome unless decompressive craniectomy is performed
- Patients with brainstem stroke generally do well and have a good rehabilitation potential
- Outcome in subarachnoid hemorrhage has improved due to increased use of endovascular coil embolization and better postprocedure care

References

1. André JM, Beis JM, Morin N, Paysant J. Buccal hemineglect. *Arch Neurol* 2000;57:1734–1741.
2. Aoun SG, Bendok BR, Batjer HH. Acute management of ruptured arteriovenous malformations and dural arteriovenous fistulas. *Neurosurg Clin N Am* 2012;23:87–103.
3. Bakheit AM, Shaw S, Carrington S, Griffiths S. The rate and extent of improvement with therapy from the different types of aphasia in the first year after stroke. *Clin Rehabil* 2007;21:941–949.
4. Balami JS, Buchan AM. Complications of intracerebral hemorrhage. *Lancet Neurol* 2012;11:101–118.
5. Bar B, Hemphill JC III. Charlson comorbidity index adjustment in intracerebral hemorrhage. *Stroke* 42:2944–2946.
6. Bath PM, Lees KR, Schellinger PD, et al. Statistical analysis of the primary outcome in acute stroke trials. *Stroke* 2012;43:1171–1178.
7. Beninato M, Gill-Body KM, Salles S, et al. Determination of the minimal clinically important difference in the FIM instrument in patients with stroke. *Arch Physa Med Relabel* 2006;87:32–39.
8. Brown RD. Simple risk predictions for arteriovenous malformation hemorrhage. *Neurosurgery* 2000;46:1024
9. Caplan LR. Scores of scores. *JAMA Neurol* 2013;70:252–253.
10. Davis SM, Broderick J, Hennerici M, et al. Hematoma growth is a determinant of mortality and poor outcome after intracerebral hemorrhage. *Neurology* 2006;66:1175–1181.
11. Duncan PW, Goldstein LB, Horner RD, et al. Similar motor recovery of upper and lower extremities after stroke. *Stroke* 1994;25:1181–1188.
12. El Hachioui H, Lingsma HF, van de Sandt-Koenderman ME, et al. Recovery of aphasia after stroke: a 1-year follow-up study. *J Neurol* 2013;260:166–171.
13. Fiehler J, Byrne JV. Factors affecting outcome after endovascular treatment of intracranial aneurysms. *Curr Opin Neurol* 2009;22:103–108.
14. Flibotte JJ, Hagan N, O'Donnell J, Greenberg SM, Rosand J. Warfarin, hematoma expansion, and outcome of intracerebral hemorrhage. *Neurology* 2004;63:1059–1064.
15. Giraldo EA, Mandrekar JN, Rubin MN, et al. Timing of clinical grade assessment and poor outcome in patients with aneurysmal subarachnoid hemorrhage. *J Neurosurg* 2012;117:15–19.
16. Greebe P, Rinkel GJ, Algra A. Long-term outcome of patients discharged to a nursing home after aneurysmal subarachnoid hemorrhage. *Arch Phys Med Rehabil* 2010;91:247–251.
17. Greebe P, Rinkel GJ, Hop JW, Visser-Meily JM, Algra A. Functional outcome and quality of life 5 and 12.5 years after aneurysmal subarachnoid hemorrhage. *J Neurol* 2010;257:2059–2064.

18. Gujjar AR, Deibert E, Manno EM, Duff S, Diringer MN. Mechanical ventilation for ischemic stroke and intracerebral hemorrhage: indications, timing, and outcome. *Neurology* 1998;51:447–451.
19. Gupta R, Connolly ES, Mayer S, Elkind MS. Hemicraniectomy for massive middle cerebral artery territory infarction: a systematic review. *Stroke* 2004;35:539–543.
20. Hop JW, Rinkel GJ, Algra A, van Gijn J. Changes in functional outcome and quality of life in patients and caregivers after aneurysmal subarachnoid hemorrhage. *J Neurosurg* 2001;95:957–963.
21. Huang J, van Gelder JM. The probability of sudden death from rupture of intracranial aneurysms: a meta-analysis. *Neurosurgery* 2002;51:1101–1105.
22. Huang P, Lin FC, Su YF, et al. Predictors of in-hospital mortality and prognosis in patients with large hemispheric stroke receiving decompressive craniectomy. *Br J Neurosurg* 2012;26:504–509.
23. Huttner HB, Kohrmann M, Berger C, Georgiadis D, Schwab S. Predictive factors for tracheostomy in neurocritical care patients with spontaneous supratentorial hemorrhage. *Cerebrovasc Dis* 2006;21:159–165.
24. Hwang BY, Appelboom G, Kellner CP, et al. Clinical grading scales in intracerebral hemorrhage. *Neurocrit Care* 2010;13:141–151.
25. Kazui S, Minematsu K, Yamamoto H, Sawada T, Yamaguchi T. Predisposing factors to enlargement of spontaneous intracerebral hematoma. *Stroke* 1997;28:2370–2375.
26. Kerkhoff G, Schenk T. Rehabilitation of neglect: an update. *Neuropsychologia* 2012;50: 1072–1079.
27. Kwakkel G, Wagenaar RC, Kollen BJ, Lankhorst GJ. Predicting disability in stroke: a critical review of the literature. *Age Ageing* 1996;25:479–489.
28. Lees KR, Bath PM, Schellinger PD, et al. Contemporary outcome measures in acute stroke research: choice of primary outcome measure. *Stroke* 2012;43:1163–1170.
29. Leira R, Dávalos A, Silva Y, et al. Early neurologic deterioration in intracerebral hemorrhage: predictors and associated factors. *Neurology* 2004;63:461–467.
30. Mahoney FI, Barthel DW. Functional evaluation: the Barthel Index. *Md State Med J* 1965;14:61–65.
31. Mauthe RW, Haaf DC, Hayn P, Krall JM. Predicting discharge destination of stroke patients using a mathematical model based on six items from the Functional Independence Measure. *Arch Phys Med Rehabil* 1996;77:10–13.
32. Mendelow AD, Gregson BA, Fernandes HM, et al. Early surgery versus initial conservative treatment in patients with spontaneous supratentorial intracerebral hematomas in the International Surgical Trial in Intracerebral Hemorrhage (STICH): a randomized trial. *Lancet* 2005;365:387–397.
33. Mendelow AD , Gregson BA , Rowan EN , Murray GD, Mitchell PM. Early surgery versus initial conservative treatment in patients with spontaneous supratentorial lobar intracerebral hematomas (STICH II): a randomized trial. *Lancet* 2013;382:397–408.
34. Navi BB, Kamel H, McCulloch CE, et al. Accuracy of neurovascular fellows' prognostication of outcome after subarachnoid hemorrhage. *Stroke* 2012;43:702–707.
35. Nijland RH, van Wegen EE, Harmeling-van der Wel BC, Kwakkel G; EPOS Investigators. Presence of finger extension and shoulder abduction within 72 hours after stroke predicts functional recovery: early prediction of functional outcome after stroke: the EPOS cohort study. *Stroke* 2010;41:745–750.
36. O'Donnell MJ, Fang J, D'Uva C, et al. The PLAN Score: a bedside prediction rule for death and severe disability following acute ischemic stroke. *Arch Intern Med* 2012;172:1580–1556.
37. Parry-Jones AR, Abid KA, Di Napoli M, et al. Accuracy and clinical usefulness of intracerebral hemorrhage grading scores: a direct comparison in a UK population. *Stroke* 2013;44:1840–1845.
38. Pradilla G, Coon AL, Huang J, Tamargo RJ. Surgical treatment of cranial arteriovenous malformations and dural arteriovenous fistulas. *Neurosurg Clin N Am* 2012;23:105–122.

39. Qureshi AI, Mendelow AD, Hanley DF. Intracerebral hemorrhage. *Lancet* 2009;373: 1632–1644.
40. Qureshi AI, Tuhrim S, Broderick JP, et al. Spontaneous intracerebral hemorrhage. *N Engl J Med* 2001;344:1450–1460.
41. Rabinstein AA, Wijdicks EFM. Determinants of outcome in anticoagulation-associated cerebral hematoma requiring emergency evacuation. *Arch Neurol* 2007;64:203–206.
42. Rabinstein AA, Wijdicks EFM. Outcome of survivors of acute stroke who require prolonged ventilatory assistance and tracheostomy. *Cerebrovasc Dis* 2004;18:325–331.
43. Rengachary J, He BJ, Shulman GL, Corbetta M. A behavioral analysis of spatial neglect and its recovery after stroke. *Front Hum Neurosci* 2011;5:29.
44. Rinkel GJ, Algra A. Long-term outcomes of patients with aneurysmal subarachnoid hemorrhage. *Lancet Neurol* 2011;10:349–356.
45. Ronkainen A, Niskanen M, Rinne J, et al. Evidence for excess long-term mortality after treated subarachnoid hemorrhage. *Stroke* 2001;32:2850–2853.
46. Rose MJ. Aneurysmal subarachnoid hemorrhage: an update on the medical complications and treatments strategies seen in these patients. *Curr Opin Anaesthesiol* 2011;24:500–507.
47. Rost NS, Smith EE, Chang Y, et al. Prediction of functional outcome in patients with primary intracerebral hemorrhage. *Stroke* 2008;39:2304–2309.
48. Stinear C. Prediction of recovery of motor function after stroke. *Lancet Neurol* 2010;9: 1228–1232.
49. The EuroQol Group. EuroQol: a new facility for the measurement of health-related quality of life. *Health Policy* 1990;16:199–208.
50. Tilley BC. Contemporary outcome measures in acute stroke research: choice of primary outcome measure and statistical analysis of the primary outcome in acute stroke trials. *Stroke* 2012;43:935–937.
51. Tuhrim S. Intracerebral hemorrhage: improving outcome by reducing volume? *N Engl J Med* 2008;358:2174–2176.
52. Uhl E, Kreth FW, Elias B, et al. Outcome and prognostic factors of hemicraniectomy for space occupying cerebral infarction. *J Neurol Neurosurg Psychiatry* 2004;75:270–274.
53. Vahedi K, Hofmeijer J, Juettler E, et al. Early decompressive surgery in malignant infarction of the middle cerebral artery: a pooled analysis of three randomized controlled trials. *Lancet Neurol* 2007;6:215–222.
54. Van Heuven AW, Dorhout Mees SM, Algra A, Rinkel GJ. Validation of a prognostic subarachnoid hemorrhage grading scale derived directly from the Glasgow Coma Scale. *Stroke* 2008;39:1347–1348.
55. Van Swieten JC, Koudstaal PJ, Visser MC, Schouten HJ, van Gijn J. Interobserver agreement for the assessment of handicap in stroke patients. *Stroke* 1988;19:604–607.
56. Visser-Meily JM, Rhebergen ML, Rinkel GJ, van Zandvoort MJ, Post MW. Long-term health-related quality of life after aneurysmal subarachnoid hemorrhage: relationship with psychological symptoms and personality characteristics. *Stroke* 2009;40:1526–1529.
57. Wermer MJ, Greebe P, Algra A, Rinkel GJ. Incidence of recurrent subarachnoid hemorrhage after clipping for ruptured intracranial aneurysms. *Stroke* 2005;36:2394–2399.
58. Wijdicks EFM, Sheth KN, Carter BS, et al. Recommendations for the management of cerebral and cerebellar infarction with swelling: a statement for healthcare professionals from the American Heart Association/American Stroke Association. *Stroke* 2014 [in press].
59. Yasaka M, Minematsu K, Naritomi H, Sakata T, Yamaguchi T. Predisposing factors for enlargement of intracerebral hemorrhage in patients treated with warfarin. *Thromb Haemost* 2003;89:278–283.

3

Prognostication After Cardiac Resuscitation

Annually, approximately 300,000 cardiac arrests occur in the United States and outside the confines of a hospital.[9,34] Cardiac arrest is usually due to a primary cardiac arrhythmia, but may also be a consequence of respiratory arrest or sudden profound hypotension. Cardiac arrest may also occur in the setting of a catastrophic acute brain injury and can be—though not invariably—an irreversible momentum.

The chance of survival, after adequate circulation has been restored, is determined by several clinical observations. Long duration of arrest—if there is evidence of a prolonged unwitnessed pulseless state or if there has been ineffective chest compression—indicates the potential of profound brain injury if the patient does not awaken. More specifically, early defibrillation has been associated with better outcome in contrast to pulseless electric activity or asystole. Number of defibrillations and use of boluses of norepinephrine or atropine also have some predictive value, but none are determinative. Still, any resuscitated patient admitted to a coronary care unit on multiple vasopressors is in an uncertain and fragile clinical state.

Survival to discharge after out-of-hospital cardiac arrest is less than 10%. When physicians are polled to estimate survival in these circumstances, the estimates are inaccurate (they are at approximately 25%); when lay persons are asked, the estimates are further off the mark (at more than 50%).[14,37] The hospital discharge rate reported in newspaper articles is twice as high as that reported in epidemiologic studies, suggesting that the public is exposed to misleading information.[15]

After the introduction of cardiopulmonary resuscitation in the early 1950s, outcome was assessed using clinical judgment alone. Even if survival was deemed unlikely or neurologic injury was expected, it did not lead to a limitation of care. At that time, prognosis in a comatose patient was often based on a single EEG or a series of studies; and when it recorded brief isoelectric intervals progressing to a near-flat EEG, outcome was judged as poor. In the 1970s and 1980s, more detailed clinical studies were performed to investigate the outcome in patients who remained comatose. One of the first observations was that an absent motor response to pain one hour after cardiopulmonary resuscitation predicted low likelihood of survival.[55] Furthermore, prospective cohorts appeared, when outcome assessment became a common reason for consulting a neurologist.[6,44–47,53,57] Sufficient clinical material has now become available, using evidence-based reviews, and allows us to separate out strong prognosticators.[51,53,61] With the frequent use of therapeutic hypothermia—an intervention considered to improve outcome in some patients—these prognosticators will have to be further examined for their value, and data is emerging that suggests there may be differences.[7,35,39]

Clinicians approaching comatose survivors after cardiac arrest have a difficult task. To incontrovertibly identify a condition that is incompatible with survival or meaningful recovery in comatose patients without brainstem injury is virtually impossible, and the ability to define the boundaries of good, not too bad, and poor outcome has proven elusive. There are many additional questions for physicians: Is it indeed possible that a minimal amount of clinical information could assist physicians in making a prediction? Could there be an exception to all these rules and what do these "outliers" mean? Should we try to identify patients who have a fighting chance? Can we be too aggressive and then simply end up with a devastated, crippled person? Perhaps most importantly resuscitation in the field and subsequent care changes over time and populations may not be easily comparable. This is true with any historical comparison but more so in this field with technology rapidly improving. This chapter discusses criteria for prognostication in postresuscitation anoxic-ischemic coma.

Principles

Before discussing the major principles of prognostication, it is useful to review the pathophysiologic changes associated with cardiac arrest and resuscitation. (other summaries can be consulted.[3,11]) The brain is able to tolerate anoxia up to 2–4 minutes, but then a process starts that results in irreversible neuronal damage. Hypoxic injury alone may result in temporary synaptic dysfunction, but with asystole, hypotension, and even the marginal cerebral perfusion during chest compression, ischemic brain injury appears. Ischemia is seen as a result of activation of the receptors of N-methyl-D-aspartate (NMDA) and α-amino-α-hydroxy-5-methyl-4-isoxazolepropionic acid (AMPA), eventually resulting in opening of calcium and sodium channels and an apoptosis pathway.[1,21] This biochemical pathway is quick and unstoppable usually in neurons that are very susceptible to anoxia–ischemic injury.

At a microscopic level, the pathology of ischemic injury involves loss of Nissl bodies, basophilia, shrinking of the perikaryon and development of triangular neurons, eosinophilia, acidophilia, and argentophilia. The pathological changes of anoxic-ischemic injury are expectedly in the watershed zones and, therefore, involve the posterior cerebral regions. With overwhelming ischemia, a complete necrosis of the cortex is seen that then also involves deeper cortical layers (laminar necrosis).

Other predilection sites include the first and second frontal gyrus (which is in a watershed zone), globus pallidus, cornu ammonis (CA) of the hippocampus, and the cerebellar cortex, predominantly the Purkinje cells. The ischemic alterations in the cornu ammonis involve the CA1 and CA4 fields. The hippocampus becomes ischemic in CA1 after several minutes of global ischemia; but necrosis occurs later, and some delayed neuronal death may occur even several days after the global ischemic insult. The CA4 region requires only minimal ischemic insult for these cells to become damaged. On the other hand, the dentate gyrus, an area that has far more proclivity for injury after hypoglycemia, is rarely involved in ischemia.

It is understood that reperfusion of ischemic tissue with oxygenated blood will activate these apoptotic mechanisms;—known as "reperfusion injury." Because reperfusion injury may be a major mechanism, there has been interest in delaying its onset at the time of resuscitation. New interest has emerged in ischemic post-conditioning.[42,64] This concept, could lead to cardiopulmonary resuscitation coupled with controlled pauses.

What has become clear is that hypothermia—when induced with artificial means—may have effects on these pathways through multiple mechanisms.[43,50,63] Hypothermia may prevent the consequences of excitotoxicity by limiting calcium influx through the AMPA channel, and may have an effect on both the intrinsic pathway (from within the cell at the level of mitochondria) and the extrinsic pathway (triggered through a self-service receptor). There is evidence that hypothermia may prevent the release of cytochrome C and may up-regulate anti-apoptotic proteins that are involved in self-survival. Hypothermia has also been documented to reduce neutrophils and inflammatory mediators such as reactive oxygen species (ROS) and reactive nitrogen species, adhesion molecules, and tumor necrosis factor.[10] Most interesting is the recent discovery that hypothermia also has an effect on the blood-brain barrier and may reduce brain edema formation by suppressing aquaporin 4 expression.[58] There is insufficient evidence that hypothermia has an effect on repair and neurogenesis.[59,60]

One of the most important core principles in prognostication of comatose patients after cardiopulmonary arrest is that it remains very difficult to predict a good outcome.[27,30,31,35] This is due to fairly rapid improvement in some patients with initially poor neurologic findings. Even pupil and corneal reflexes may return after blood pressure is restored to consistently normal levels. Therefore, most studies have concentrated on finding indicators of poor prognosis and low likelihood of improvement. It remains important to recognize that the brainstem is typically spared. This indicates that absent pupillary or corneal reflexes are much less common, and that in most patients the motor response to noxious stimuli might be the best indicator of the degree of cortical injury.[62]

Any prediction has now been challenged by therapeutic hypothermia that has improved outcome in these patients. If a new therapy improves outcome, the prognostic factors may change, though not necessarily. Certain findings could remain indicative of permanent damage no matter what the intervention. Moreover, certain therapies may add new confounders, which is exactly the case with therapeutic hypothermia. Therapeutic hypothermia requires the use of sedatives, neuromuscular blockers, and analgesics, and doses used vary considerably. Moreover, anoxic-ischemic injury to the brain rarely damages the brain alone. The lingering cumulative effects of these drugs in patients with resuscitation-associated renal and liver injury may additionally make a neurologic examination less reliable.

In Practice

Outcome assessment after cardiopulmonary resuscitation has now evolved into prognostication after therapeutic hypothermia and prognostication without therapeutic hypothermia. This distinction is justified knowing that this intervention improves outcome, albeit modestly. Utilization of therapeutic hypothermia protocols is variable but increasing worldwide. In fact, the range is still very wide, with estimates of patients treated with therapeutic hypothermia in the 20%–90% bracket. In a recent U.S./Canadian trial testing an impedance threshold device in out-of-hospital cardiac arrest, 47% of over 4,000 patients in 10 sites received therapeutic hypothermia.[2]

We will first discuss prognosis of patients not treated with therapeutic hypothermia. The American Academy of Neurology (AAN) has outlined practice guidelines based on prehypothermia data. Unfortunately, few studies were available that could be assessed accurately; and a large number of studies lacked both a detailed clinical examination and a clearly defined poor outcome. The reliability of the data used in the AAN guidelines was further set as a false-positive rate of 0 with a narrow confidence interval. Thus, the false positive rate in this context is best understood as the number of instances that the outcome is better than poor despite the test indicating a poor outcome. (Ideally this number is zero or close to zero.)

In any patient who is assessed for outcome, confounders need to be examined carefully. If none of these confounders are present, a combination of laboratory tests—particularly serum neuron-specific enolase (NSE) and somatosensory evoked potentials (SSEP)—and clinical findings such as myoclonic status epilepticus, absent pupil and corneal reflexes, and absent motor responses to a noxious stimulus 72 hours from arrest are reliable predictors. Absent pupillary responses and a mid-position pupil with absent corneal reflexes and absent oculocephaic responses could be particularly indicative of a poor outcome and are a reflection of a far more severe injury damaging the brainstem, but such details are not often found in recent series of patients.[52,53]

How can we proceed with prognostication in a patient who has been treated with therapeutic hypothermia? Until very recently it has been the understanding that therapeutic hypothermia has improved outcome of patients resuscitated after out-of-hospital cardiac arrest, but the intervention has only been proven in patients with shockable rhythms, not in patients with asystole or pulseless electrical activity.[4,22,28] Some studies claim there might still be a positive effect in these patients as well, and practices now often subject these patients to this intervention.[24,28]

Cooling of the patient implies achieving a core temperature of 32°C–33°C; this intervention has improved outcome to 55% in the hypothermia group compared with 39% in the control group in prior studies. This beneficial effect has been recently challenged by two clinical trials. One showed prehospital cooling did not improve outcome and the other found no benefit comparing 33°C with 36°C. These clinical trials seriously question the claimed benefit of "therapeutic" hypothermia and may change practice to fever control only.[23,29]

Most studies have evaluated prognosis at 72 hours after cardiopulmonary resuscitation treated with therapeutic hypothermia.[18–20,24] One of the first studies of prognostication after therapeutic hypothermia found imperfect FPR for known prognosticators: myoclonus (3% FPR) no motor response to pain (24% FPR), and even added incomplete recovery of brainstem reflexes (4% FPR).[39] Serum NSE, initially found to be an independent predictor in at least three studies, is not maintaining its predictive value in patients treated with hypothermia. However, absent N20 responses on SSEP remains highly predictive after use of therapeutic hypothermia.[5,7,8,18] A guide for prognostication in anoxic-ischemic coma is provided in Figure 3.1.

Rather than doing a "spot EEG" and repeating it for comparison, as was a common practice in the distant past, there has been renewed interest in EEG monitoring.[48] In the prehypothermia era, the AAN evidence-based guideline found insufficient data to conclude that certain EEG patterns to be definitively prognosticating.

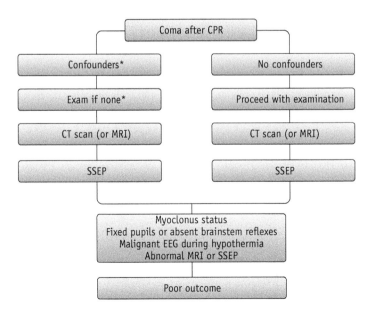

Figure 3.1 Predicting factors of prognosis after cardiopulmonary resuscitation.
* sedatives, analgesics, neuromuscular blockers, hypothermia.

In recent years there has been a surge of continuous EEG (cEEG) monitoring in these patients. cEEG has been recommended during therapeutic hypothermia to provide prognostic information and to monitor for subclinical seizures.[25,35] Another justification for using cEEG is that hypothermia may reduce seizures or change EEG abnormalities, and in experimental studies has antiepileptic effects. Conversely, the risk of seizures can increase during rewarming.

It has been found that seizures detected on cEEG during therapeutic hypothermia often are associated with unreactive backgrounds and discontinuous patterns and, when found in comatose patients, the outcome is poor.[38-41] However, it should be noted that reactivity (i.e., reactivity to light or pain stimulus) is greatly affected by sedation, analgesia, and perhaps even by therapeutic hypothermia. Other patterns, such as the presence of diffuse slow wave activity in the absence of malignant patterns such as burst suppression or generalized periodic epileptiform discharges (GPEDs), correlate with a better prognosis. Common EEG patterns are shown in Figure 3.2.

In our experience, nearly three-quarters of patients have the same EEG pattern during therapeutic hypothermia, rewarming, and normothermia. Other than diffuse background slowing, the most common EEG finding are episodic low amplitude events (ELAEs).[12] ELAEs can be associated with medication effects and thus are not necessarily indicative of hypoxic-ischemic cerebral injury.

Background EEG activity that demonstrates generalized slow wave activity more often predicts a good outcome.[23] A burst suppression pattern is more often associated with fatal outcome or vegetative state. It generally can be said that the presence of faster EEG frequency with spontaneous fluctuation and reactivity to stimuli does indicate a possible neurologic recovery.

Some patients have diffuse epileptiform discharges, also known as periodic lateralized epileptiform discharges (PLEDs), bilateral independent PLEDs (BIPLEDs) or generalized periodic epileptiform discharges (GPEDs.) These interictal patterns do not necessarily indicate a poor outcome. Whether GPEDS are seizures is controversial, and many experts consider them interictal, particularly when consistently ≥2 or 2.5 Hz.[35] GPEDS do indicate a higher susceptibility to seizures.

Treating seizures after cardiopulmonary resuscitation may need to be better established if cEEG is recommended to detect seizures. There may even be a discussion on what should be considered a seizure.[33,35] In our patients, malignant background patterns are often present prior to the onset of seizures. Most studies have found that patients who had clinical seizures remained comatose and died from withdrawal of support irrespective of treatment. In summary, with the emergence of cEEG, new interesting findings have come to light; however, there is no clear guidance on how to interpret the EEG findings and how to use them in prognosticating. One could prudently conclude that seizures during therapeutic hypothermia are a poor sign, seizures after rewarming may be a poor sign but could be treated if arising from a reactive background, and seizures with an abnormal SSEP, CT or MRI could be a poor sign as well.

Another issue is the reliability of serum NSE, a well-recognized biomarker of hypoxic-ischemic brain injury. Prior studies have found a cutoff of 33 ng/mL, above

Anesthetic pattern

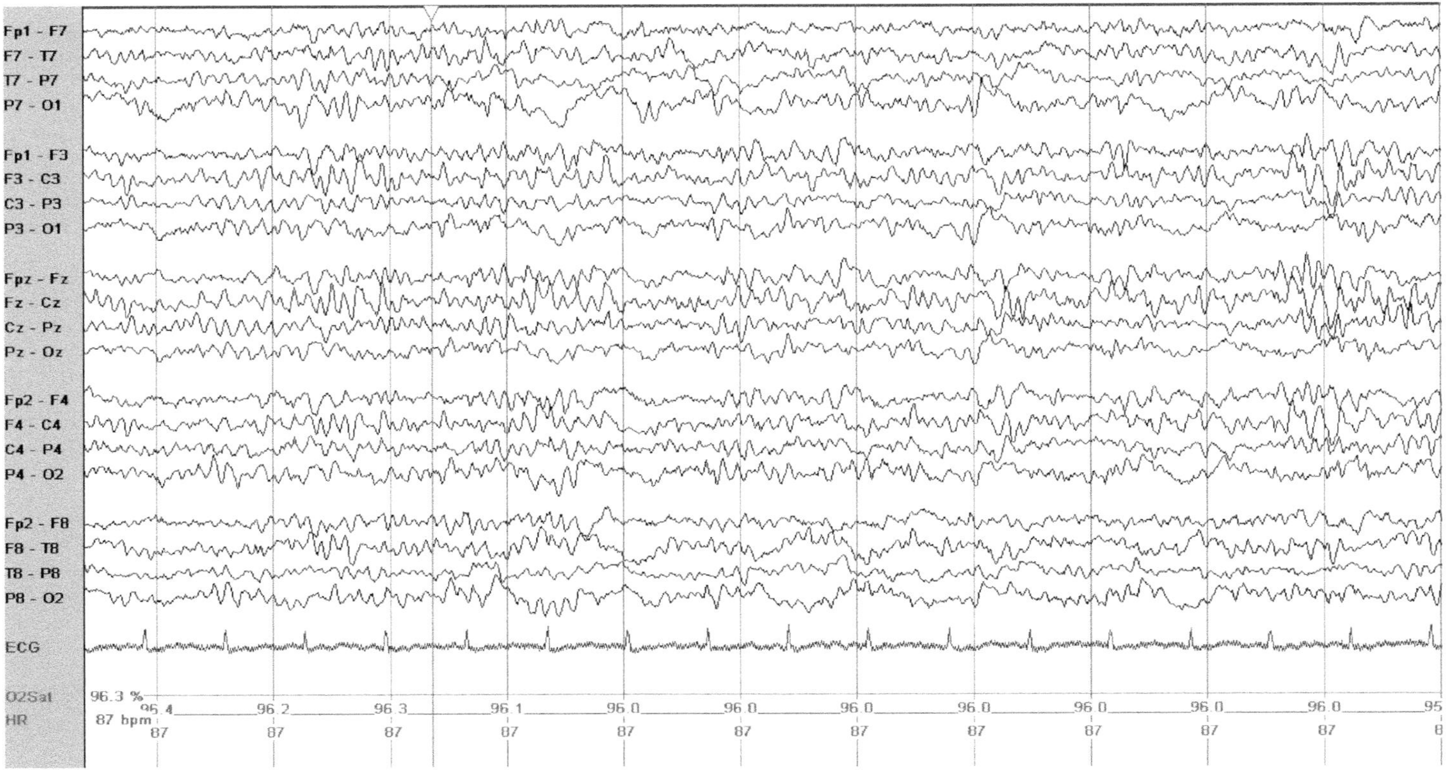

Figure 3.2 Common EEG Patterns After Cardiac Arrest.

Diffuse Delta Pattern

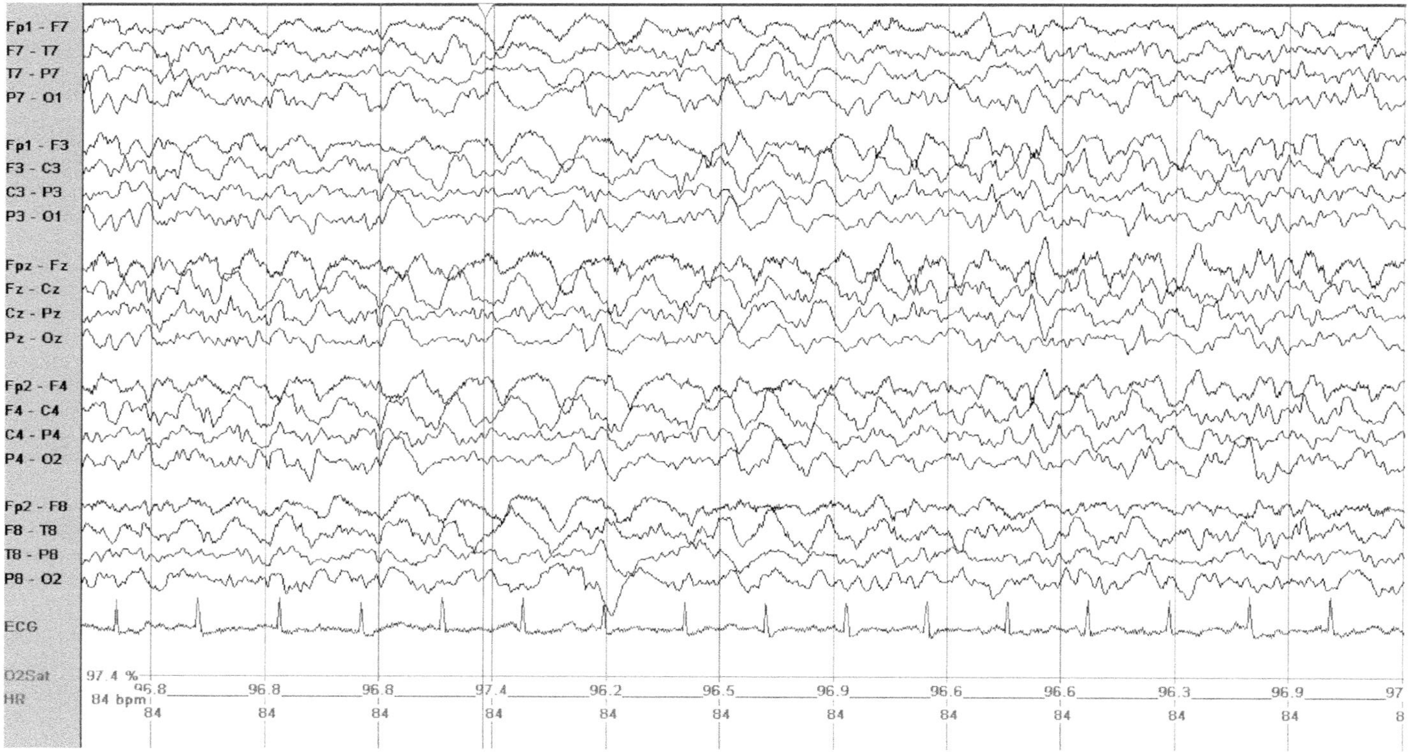

Figure 3.2 (Continued)

Episodic Low Amplitude Event

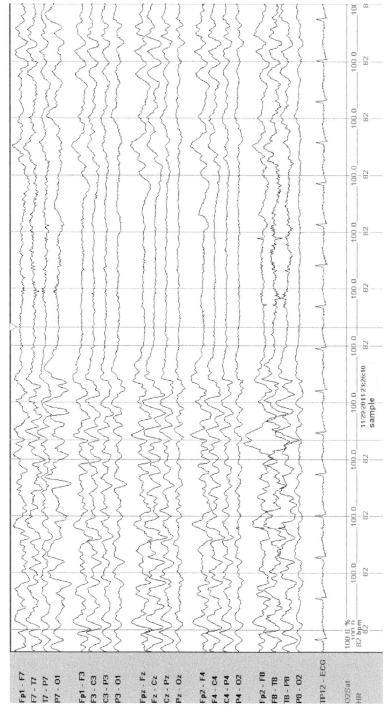

Figure 3.2 (Continued)

Generalized Electrographic Seizure Preceded by Burst Suppression Background

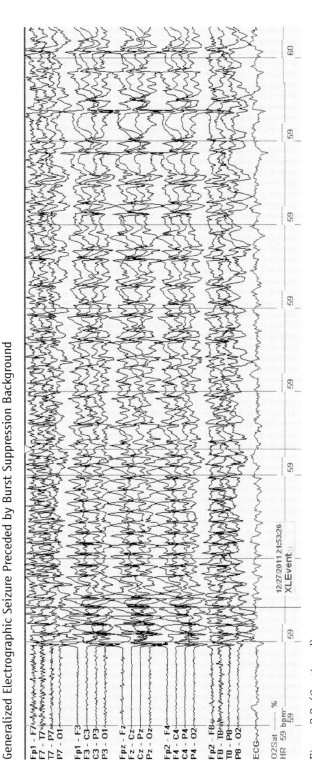

Figure 3.2 (Continued)

which injury is more likely. However again, the value of serum NSE after therapeutic hypothermia is much less clear and multiple studies have found no correlation between NSE in treated patients and outcome. A higher NSE cutoff value might be a better prognostication.[13] (The cutoff value of NSE in one study was 97 ng/mL and had a 100% positive predictive value for poor outcome.) Poor outcome was more likely if NSE was combined with malignant EEG patterns or absent SSEPs.[13]

It would be ill advised to make decisions based on one laboratory test, particularly because in one study of 36 patients with an absent N20 on SSEP, 1 patient survived with normal neurologic outcome (not finding a N20 response may be a technical flaw).[26]

Most CT scans are normal at the time of cardiac arrest, but follow-up CT scans days later may become abnormal. Most damaging and concerning is the emergence of diffuse brain edema, but many of these patients already have clinical features suggesting a poor outcome. One study found that the ratio of median Hounsfield units in the putamen to the posterior lip of the internal capsule predicted poor outcome.[56] Much more predictive for outcome is MRI, which may detect diffuse cortical injury that may involve bithalamic and putaminal regions.[49,54,57] A normal MRI scan cannot be seen as a good prognostic sign, because we have seen several patients in a persistent vegetative state or minimally conscious state with repeatedly normal MRI scans who showed more brain atrophy in the months thereafter.

The determination of poor outcome is difficult; when practices are audited, it appears that poor prognosis may not always be well documented, and patients may have even had their care withdrawn while undergoing hypothermia.[32] The reason for withdrawal of care is not always clear in patients in coronary care units, and not all patients are necessarily seen by a neurologist. How laboratory tests influence the decision to withdraw care has also not been adequately investigated, and relevant data would be difficult to obtain. Often these patients are on multiple vasopressors with associated kidney and renal dysfunction or progressive cardiovascular collapse. In some patients, terminal cardiac failure is just overwhelming, so neurologic assessment takes a back seat and in fact may not contribute much.

Finally, very few studies have carefully looked into abnormalities of cognitive domains of survivors following therapeutic hypothermia. In a recent study at Mayo Clinic, approximately 40% of patients had memory and attention difficulties, but the majority of patients returned to work.[16]

By the Way

- Drugs administered during hypothermia may have a prolonged effect
- Treatment of myoclonus status does not improve outcome
- CT scan with severe brain edema is uncommon after CPR
- Treatment of brain edema after cardiac arrest and CPR is not helpful
- Neuroimaging may be normal in patients with poor outcome

Coma After Cardiac Arrest by the Numbers

- ~100% of patients in post resuscitation PVS for one year remain in PVS
- ~75% of patients with in-hospital arrest survive to discharge
- ~60% of comatose patients have no cognitive deficits
- ~10% of patients with out-of-hospital arrest survive to discharge
- ~5% of comatose patients after CPR become brain dead

Putting It All Together

- Clinical features of the neurologic examination may be markedly suppressed by drugs used during hypothermia, and effects may linger
- Damage to the brainstem, with absent pupil and corneal reflexes, is a major guiding principle to determine outcome
- It is still not clear whether epileptiform activity or seizures in comatose patients after cardiopulmonary resuscitation are treatable complications or manifestations of a severely damaged cortex
- Malignant EEG patterns during hypothermia are poor prognostic factors

References

1. Andrabi SA, Dawson TM, Dawson VL. Mitochondrial and nuclear cross talk in cell death: parthanatos. *Ann N Y Acad Sci* 2008;1147:233–241.
2. Aufderheide TP, Nichols G, Rea TD, et al. A trial of an impedance device in out-of-hospital cardiac arrest. *N Engl J Med*.2011;365:798–806.
3. Ayoub IM, Radhakrishnan J, Gazmuri RJ. Targeting mitochondria for resuscitation from cardiac arrest. *Crit Care Med* 2008;36:S440–S446.
4. Bernard SA, Gray TW, Buist MD, et al. Treatment of comatose survivors of out-of-hospital cardiac arrest with induced hypothermia. *N Engl J Med* 2002;346:557–563.
5. Bisschops LL, van Alfen N, Bons S, van der Hoeven JG, Hoedemaekers CW. Predictors of poor neurologic outcome in patients after cardiac arrest treated with hypothermia: a retrospective study. *Resuscitation* 2011;82: 696–701.
6. Booth CM, Boone RH, Tomlinson G, Detsky AS. Is this patient dead, vegetative, or severely neurologically impaired? Assessing outcome for comatose survivors of cardiac arrest. *JAMA* 2004;291:870–879.
7. Bouwes A, Binnekade JM, Kuiper MA, et al. Prognosis of coma after therapeutic hypothermia: a prospective cohort study. *Ann Neurol* 2012;71:206–212.
8. Bouwes A, Binnekade JM, Zandstra DF, et al. Somatosensory evoked potentials during mild hypothermia after cardiopulmonary resuscitation. *Neurology* 2009;73:1457–1461.
9. Bunch TJ, White RD, Gersh BJ, et al. Long-term outcomes of out-of-hospital cardiac arrest after successful early defibrillation. *N Engl J Med* 2003;348:2626–2633.
10. Colbourne F, Li H, Buchan AM. Indefatigable CA1 sector neuroprotection with mild hypothermia induced 6 hours after severe forebrain ischemia in rats. *J Cereb Blood Flow Metab* 1999;19:742–749.

11. Cour M, Gomez L, Mewton N, Ovize M, Argaud L. Postconditioning: from the bench to bedside. *J Cardiovasc Pharmacol Ther* 2011;16:117–130.

12. Crepeau AZ, Rabinstein AA, Fugate JE, et al. Continuous EEG in therapeutic hypothermia after cardiac arrest: prognostic and clinical value. *Neurology* 2013;80:339–344.

13. Daubin C, Quentin C, Allouche S, et al. Serum neuron-specific enolase as predictor of outcome in comatose cardiac-arrest survivors: a prospective cohort study. *BMC Cardiovasc Disord* 2011;11:48.

14. Donohoe RT, Haefeli K, Moore F. Public perceptions and experiences of myocardial infarction, cardiac arrest and CPR in London. *Resuscitation* 2006;71:70–79.

15. Field RA, Soar J, Nolan JP, Perkins GD. Epidemiology and outcome of cardiac arrests reported in the lay-press: an observational study. *J R Soc Med* 2011;104:525–531.

16. Fugate JE, Moore A, Knopman DS, Claassen DO, Wijdicks EFM, Rabinstein AA. Cognitive outcome of patients under going therapeutic hypothermia after cardiac arrest. *Neurology* 2013;81:40–45.

17. Fugate JE, Rabinstein AA, Claassen DO, White RD, Wijdicks EFM. The FOUR score predicts outcome in patients after cardiac arrest. *Neurocrit Care* 2010;13:205–210.

18. Fugate JE, Wijdicks EFM, Mandrekar J, et al. Predictors of neurologic outcome in hypothermia after cardiac arrest. *Ann Neurol* 2010;68:907–914.

19. Fugate JE, Wijdicks EFM, White RD, Rabinstein AA. Does therapeutic hypothermia affect time to awakening in cardiac arrest survivors? *Neurology* 2011;77:1346–1350.

20. Geocadin RG, Kaplan PW. Neural repair and rehabilitation: the effect of therapeutic hypothermia on prognostication. *Nat Rev Neurol* 2011;8:5–6.

21. Green DR, Reed JC. Mitochondria and apoptosis. *Science* 1998;281:1309–1312.

22. Hypothermia After Cardiac Arrest Study Group. Mild therapeutic hypothermia to improve the neurologic outcome after cardiac arrest. *N Engl J Med* 2002;346:549–556.

23. Kim F, Nichol G, Maynard C, et al. Effect of prehospital induction of hypothermia on survival and neurological status among adults with cardiac arrest: a randomized clinical trial. *JAMA* 2014;311:45–52.

24. Kawai M, Thapalia U, Verma A. Outcome from therapeutic hypothermia and EEG. *J Clin Neurophysiol* 2011;28:483–488.

25. Legriel S, Bruneel F, Sediri H, et al. Early EEG monitoring for detecting postanoxic status epilepticus during therapeutic hypothermia: a pilot study. *Neurocrit Care* 2009;11:338–344.

26. Leithner C, Ploner CJ, Hasper D, Storm C. Does hypothermia influence the predictive value of bilateral absent N20 after cardiac arrest? *Neurology* 2010;74:965–969.

27. Levy DE, Caronna JJ, Singer BH, Lapinski RH, Frydman H, Plum F. Predicting outcome from hypoxic-ischemic coma. *JAMA* 1985;253:1420–1426.

28. Lundbye JB, Rai M, Ramu B, et al. Therapeutic hypothermia is associated with improved neurologic outcome and survival in cardiac arrest survivors of non-shockable rhythms. *Resuscitation* 2012;83:202–207.

29. Nielsen N, Wetterslev J, Cronberg T, et al. Targeted temperature management at 33°C versus 36°C after cardiac arrest. *N Engl J Med* 2013;369:2197–2206.

30. Nolan JP, Laver SR, Welch CA, et al. Outcome following admission to UK intensive care units after cardiac arrest: a secondary analysis of the ICNARC Case Mix Programme Database. *Anaesthesia* 2007;62:1207–1216.

31. Nolan JP, Neumar RW, Adrie C, et al. Post-cardiac arrest syndrome: epidemiology, pathophysiology, treatment, and prognostication: a scientific statement from the International Liaison Committee on Resuscitation; the American Heart Association Emergency Cardiovascular Care Committee; the Council on Cardiovascular Surgery and Anesthesia; the Council on Cardiopulmonary, Perioperative, and Critical Care; the Council on Clinical Cardiology; the Council on Stroke. *Resuscitation* 2008;79:350–379.

32. Perman SM, Kirkpatrick JN, Reitsma AM, et al. Timing of neuroprognostication in postcardiac arrest therapeutic hypothermia. *Crit Care Med* 2012;40:719–724.

33. Rabinstein AA, Wijdicks EFM. The value of EEG monitoring after cardiac arrest treated with hypothermia. *Neurology* 2012;78:774–775.

34. Rea TD, Pearce RM, Raghunathan TE, et al. Incidence of out-of-hospital cardiac arrest. *Am J Cardiol* 2004;93:1455–1460.

35. Rittenberger JC, Popescu A, Brenner RP, Guyette FX, Callaway CW. Frequency and timing of nonconvulsive status epilepticus in comatose post-cardiac arrest subjects treated with hypothermia. *Neurocrit Care* 2012;16:114–122.

36. Rittenberger JC, Sangl J, Wheeler M, Guyette FX, Callaway CW. Association between clinical examination and outcome after cardiac arrest. *Resuscitation* 2010;81:1128–1132.

37. Roberts D, Hirschman D, Scheltema K. Adult and pediatric CPR: attitudes and expectations of health professionals and laypersons. *Am J Emerg Med* 2000;18:465–468.

38. Rossetti AO, Carrera E, Oddo M. Early EEG correlates of neuronal injury after brain anoxia. *Neurology* 2012;78:796–802.

39. Rossetti AO, Oddo M, Logroscino G, Kaplan PW. Prognostication after cardiac arrest and hypothermia: a prospective study. *Ann Neurol* 2010;67:301–307.

40. Rossetti AO, Urbano LA, Delodder F, Kaplan PW, Oddo M. Prognostic value of continuous EEG monitoring during therapeutic hypothermia after cardiac arrest. *Crit Care* 2010;14:R173.

41. Rundgren M, Westhall E, Cronberg T, Rosén I, Friberg H. Continuous amplitude-integrated electroencephalogram predicts outcome in hypothermia-treated cardiac arrest patients. *Crit Care Med* 2010;38:1838–1844.

42. Segal N, Matsuura T, Caldwell E, et al. Ischemic postconditioning at the initiation of cardiopulmonary resuscitation facilitates functional cardiac and cerebral recovery after prolonged untreated ventricular fibrillation. *Resuscitation* 2012;83:1397–1403.

43. Silasi G, Colbourne F. Therapeutic hypothermia influences cell genesis and survival in the rat hippocampus following global ischemia. *J Cereb Blood Flow Metab* 2011;31:1725–1735.

44. Snyder BD, Gumnit RJ, Leppik IE, Hauser A, Loewenson RB, Ramirez-Lassepas M. Neurologic prognosis after cardiopulmonary arrest. IV. Brainstem reflexes. *Neurology* 1981;31:1092–1097.

45. Snyder BD, Hauser A, Loewenson RB, Leppik IE, Ramirez-Lassepas M, Gumnit RJ. Neurologic prognosis after cardiopulmonary arrest. III. Seizure activity. *Neurology* 1980;30:1292–1297.

46. Snyder BD, Loewenson RB, Gumnit RJ, Hauser A, Leppik IE, Ramirez-Lassepas M. Neurologic prognosis after cardiopulmonary arrest. II. level of consciousness. *Neurology* 1980;30:52–58.

47. Snyder BD, Ramirez-Lassepas M, Lippert DM. Neurologic status and prognosis after cardiopulmonary arrest. I. a retrospective study. *Neurology* 1977;27:807–811.

48. Thenayan EA, Savard M, Sharpe MD, Norton L, Young B. Electroencephalogram for prognosis after cardiac arrest. *J Crit Care* 2010;25:300–304.

49. Torbey MT, Bhardwaj A. MR imaging in comatose survivors of cardiac resuscitation. *AJNR Am J Neuroradiol* 2002;23:738.

50. Webster CM, Kelly S, Koike MA, et al. Inflammation and NFkappaB activation is decreased by hypothermia following global cerebral ischemia. *Neurobiol Dis* 2009;33:301–312.

51. Wijdicks EFM. From clinical judgment to odds: a history of prognostication in anoxic coma. *Resuscitation* 2012;83:940–945.

52. Wijdicks EFM, Parisi JE, Sharbrough FW. Prognostic value of myoclonus status in comatose survivors of cardiac arrest. *Ann Neurol* 1994;35:239–243.

53. Wijdicks EFM, Young B. Practice parameter: prediction of outcome in comatose survivors after cardiopulmonary resuscitation (an evidence-based review): report of the Quality Standards Subcommittee of the American Academy of Neurology. *Neurology* 2006;67:203–210.

54. Wijman CA, Mlynash M, Caulfield AF, et al. Prognostic value of brain diffusion-weighted imaging after cardiac arrest. *Ann Neurol* 2009;65:394–402.

55. Willoughby JO, Leach BG. Relation of neurological findings after cardiac arrest to outcome. *BMJ* 1974;3:437–439.

56. Wu O, Batista LM, Lima FO, et al. Predicting clinical outcome in comatose cardiac arrest patients using early noncontrast computed tomography. *Stroke* 2011;42:985–992.

57. Wu O, Sorensen AG, Benner T, et al. Comatose patients with cardiac arrest: predicting clinical outcome with diffusion-weighted MR imaging. *Radiology* 2009;252:173–181.

58. Xiao F, Arnold TC, Zhang S, et al. Cerebral cortical aquaporin-4 expression in brain edema following cardiac arrest in rats. *Acad Emerg Med* 2004;11:1001–1007.

59. Yenari MA, Han HS. Neuroprotective mechanisms of hypothermia in brain ischaemia. *Nat Rev Neurosci* 2012;13:267–278.

60. Yenari MA, Liu J, Zheng Z, Vexler ZS, Lee JE, Giffard RG. Antiapoptotic and anti-inflammatory mechanisms of heat-shock protein protection. *Ann N Y Acad Sci* 2005;1053:74–83.

61. Zandbergen EG, de Haan RJ, Stoutenbeek CP, Koelman JH, Hijdra A. Systematic review of early prediction of poor outcome in anoxic-ischemic coma. *Lancet* 1998;352:1808–1812.

62. Zandbergen EG, Hijdra A, Koelman JH, et al. Prediction of poor outcome within the first 3 days of postanoxic coma. *Neurology* 2006;66:62–68.

63. Zhang H, Zhou M, Zhang J, et al. Initiation time of post-ischemic hypothermia on the therapeutic effect in cerebral ischemic injury. *Neural Res.* 2009;31:336–339.

64. Zhao H. Ischemic postconditioning as a novel avenue to protect against brain injury after stroke. *J Cereb Blood Flow Metab* 2009;29:873–885.

4

Prognostication after Seizures or Status Epilepticus

Outcome after a single seizure depends on the type of seizure and whether the seizure is provoked and by what. To predict the time course of seizures in acute brain injury—that is, anticipating recurrence and even anticipating progression to status epilepticus—depends on many factors and thus is nearly an impossible task.

Outcome of unprovoked or provoked seizures is different from provoked seizures associated with acute brain injury. The long-term recurrence rate of unprovoked seizures is still approximately 50%.[17] On the other hand, the recurrence rate can be low in provoked seizures if the cause is drug intoxication or an acute metabolic derangement.

Outcome in seizures is also determined by factors such as compliance with antiepileptic agents (generally poor); elimination of provoking factors such as alcohol abuse (not much better), certain antidepressants, or psychotropic agents (few alternative options); and type of drug used (some drugs provide much better control of partial seizures than others).

The outcome is also much different in patients with a rapid succession of seizures. Typically patients with a flurry of seizures do just fine (assuming no other major neurologic illness) but most patients in status epilepticus do not do well. Precise definition of status epilepticus is a problem, and thus precise definition of outcome is a problem. Etiologies for status epilepticus are quite diverse—in the vast majority no etiology can be found. The most common causes for status epilepticus in adults includes chronic epilepsy, brain tumor, neurodegenerative disease, traumatic head injury and prior alcoholism, central nervous system (CNS) infection stroke and acute metabolic causes. Furthermore, the treatment approach used may impact outcome. Any physician accepts that there is one important observation in these patients—time to treatment of status epilepticus matters. It is also a reality that some patients are treated late and inappropriately, which affects outcome. Once the patient in status epilepticus is treated with multiple antiepileptic drugs and has not been responding to traditional IV (fos)phenytoin loading and several doses of long-acting benzodiazepines, it becomes immediately clear that outcome may be compromised. Long-term management of status epilepticus with multiple unsuccessful attempts at lowering the medication is always associated with systemic complications and even temporary life-threatening situations requiring resuscitation.

Prognostication of status epilepticus is difficult. In some ways, the true nature of the disorder can only be appreciated after several weeks. That some patients may be able to pull themselves out of this state is nothing more than a surprise, but every physician working in the field has noted a good outcome in some patients who initially appear not to respond well to treatment.[32,50]

So what are the questions to ask after a flurry of seizures? What if we cannot treat incessant seizures? When is outcome assessment warranted or justified? What is the broader issue when seizures keep returning? This chapter discusses the current available evidence of prognostic factors that impact morbidity and mortality after status epilepticus.

Principles

Several pieces of information are needed, at the least including how the seizures were generated. Putting aside the biologic changes associated with continuous seizures, in some patients seizures may be very difficult to detect or may remain unrecognized if an abnormal response is attributed to other causes. It is safe to say that seizures in comatose patients (particularly nonconvulsive seizures) are underdiagnosed.

Any acute brain lesion may cause seizures, but there are different mechanisms. Seizures after an ischemic stroke are a consequence of direct irritability of the cortex. These cortical lesions may become an epileptic focus and may spread into other cortical areas, perhaps during evolution of the ischemic penumbra. However, there appears to be reduction of depolarization when ischemic tissue becomes necrotic. (In experimental settings, blocking these action potentials early may reduce seizures.[16]) Late seizures may be a consequence of gliosis. Conversely, one can expect a near-virtual absence of seizures with lacunar strokes.[17]

The pathophysiology of seizures in intracerebral hemorrhage may be different and related to thrombin. Although under the cortex, the damage of white matter (i.e., lobar hematoma) could result in a hyperexcitable cortex through pressure effects. In experimental studies thrombin is epileptogenic and such a mechanism has been proven by stopping seizures with a thrombin inhibitor.[25]

The genesis of seizures in traumatic brain injury may be due to a complex interplay of factors. Glial scars, neuronal disruption, and reduction of inhibitory neurons have been proposed as factors that increase seizure development. Ionic homeostasis may be disturbed and is supported by experimental studies showing abnormal potassium traffic in hippocampal slices.[8]

There are several important principles. A first core principle is that there is generally a brief time window where treatment could be effective, but there are also patients in whom basically nothing works and physicians quickly run out of options. Procrastination in treatment of status epilepticus will result in more-difficult-to-control status epilepticus.[12] This is a result of both changes of the GABAergic receptor function (see volume *Handling Difficult Situations*) and possibly mitochondrial changes in the neuron itself. Early studies have found that even seizure duration of an hour or more is an important determinant of outcome.[10,11] A second core principle is that status epilepticus should be divided into nonconvulsive status epilepticus, convulsive status epilepticus, myoclonus status epilepticus, and—a quite common form—focal status epilepticus.[23,24,26,45] Each of these disorders has a different outcome, and most of it is determined by the initial response to antiepileptic drugs.

A third core principle is that there are untreatable neurologic disorders such as recurrent glioblastoma, late diagnosis of a destructive CNS infection, or global anoxic-ischemic injury after cardiopulmonary resuscitation that will make a successful outcome practically impossible.[39] Some young patients with no prior illness or seizure disorder may develop refractory status epilepticus with no apparent cause even after multiple (viral, toxicological, immunological, paraneoplastic, and genetic) tests. This condition, termed new-onset refractory status epilepticus (NORSE), may be associated with a mild lymphocytic pleocytosis and emerging MRI abnormalities that could be attributed to the seizures themselves. Outcome has been poor in most cases, and autopsy has always been unrevealing and frustratingly nonspecific.[7]

A fourth core principle is that the prognosis is obviously determined by the way the patient is treated.[9,31,40-42] The methodology to obtain adequate data in status epilepticus may be far from perfect.[31] The condition of patients with multiple unsuccessful treatments is now called super-refractory status epilepticus. This new classification may have value only if it can be clearly delineated from refractory status epilepticus, and that is not yet the case. Furthermore, it is possible that rapid and early weaning of anesthetics may be associated with high rates of recurrence and may cause additional neuronal stress, but very little data exists. Even the degree to which electrographically recordings are suppressed may play a role. It is unclear whether burst suppression or prolonged periods of silent EEG are required in all or certain cases. It is also not known if in patients with already demonstrated recurrence after weaning, a more aggressive suppression of the EEG background may be more effective.

In Practice

Acute brain injury increases the probability of focal or generalized seizures. There is sufficient evolving evidence that 24- to 48-hour monitoring in stuporous patients with acute brain injury detects more seizures or epileptiform foci. Whether periodic epileptiform discharges (PEDs) are clinically important is not known, because nonspecific conditions such as sepsis and renal failure may already change EEG without clinical consequences.[37] Treatment of nonconvulsive EEG patterns may improve outcome only if prior seizures have been noted clinically.[43]

APPROACHING SINGLE (OR A FEW MORE) SEIZURES

Seizures after acute brain injury in hospitalized patients can be seen in strikingly diverse clinical circumstances. It is ultimately important to quickly find the cause but also to consider the possibility of another trigger. For example, a patient with a subdural hematoma may have developed severe hyponatremia or may have been recently started on an antibiotic such as imipenem or cephalosporin.

What can we expect to see in the hospital, and what are the more acute conditions? First, seizures may occur with drugs of abuse, but seizures are uncommon in intoxications and far less frequent than pharmacy textbooks suggest. Psychotropic drugs have been notoriously cited as triggers for seizures, but this is not that common. If an association is sought, it may be found in the use of large doses of antidepressants, mostly selective serotonin reuptake inhibitors (SSRIs) and lithium. SSRI's can cause a serotonin syndrome marked by myoclonus or seizures and extreme rigidity. With lithium overdose fasciculations and cerebellar dysfunction, but also choreiform movements are part of the clinical manifestation. This is rapidly followed by seizures and coma when the serum levels reach 3.5 mEq/L.

Second, seizures can be expected in critically ill patients with metabolic shifts and electrolyte abnormalities, as a result of either drug toxicity or a specific medical illness. Acute metabolic derangements that may often cause recurrent seizures are hypoglycemia and hyponatremia. Hypoglycemia almost always results from insulin overdose. Tonic-clonic seizures associated with hypoglycemia may be focal, but typically become generalized. Prompt treatment in patients with suspected hypoglycemia raises blood levels quickly, and seizures then stop.

Dilutional hyponatremia is a very common electrolyte disturbance in hospitalized surgical patients. A sudden decrease in serum sodium concentration—a major downward shift of 20 mmol/L, and often less than 110 mmol/L—is needed to cause a seizure. If a seizure is associated with an acute metabolic derangement that can be quickly corrected, it is reasonable to hold back antiepileptic drugs while correcting the metabolic derangement. However, when there are recurrent seizures, and time to correction is deliberately slow—as in hyponatremia—intravenous administration of phenytoin or fosphenytoin (20 mg/kg) or levetiracetam (1,000–2,000 mg IV load) is warranted to bridge the period during which the metabolic derangement is corrected. However, prognosis for recovery often remains uncertain, and is frequently poor in patients with seizures associated with acute metabolic changes, largely because of the underlying illness causing the derangement.

Transplant recipients with acute seizures are a separate category. Immunosuppressive agents, such as cyclosporine and tacrolimus, and antibiotics given prophylactically should be first excluded as major causes. Any new seizure in a transplant recipient could foretell a major medical or neurologic problem. Seizures have been reported frequently in liver transplant recipients, and in some series may have been seen in 10% to 20% of patients. Seizures may also occur in patients with a rapidly evolving rejection of the liver graft. This is recognized by increasing arterial ammonia and is a major problem in itself, impacting on survival of the patient. In the early days of transplantation, seizures were associated with neuro-toxicity—this now seems much less common—but it should remain a consideration in any patient with a liver transplant. Other less common causes are acute hyponatremia, hypomagnesemia, and hyperglycemia, but all published information is poorly detailed and seizures have usually been linked to neurotoxicity.

Management of seizures in transplant recipients typically involves an anti-epileptic drug, even if there has been a single seizure and for certain if there is a structural lesion. The reason to be so aggressive and preemptive is that a seizure is a major medical challenge to these fragile patients. If antiepileptic drugs are considered, intravenous levetiracetam is probably the best agent to use, and the least hepatotoxic.

A now better-recognized cause of seizures is when patients have prior labile hypertension and a posterior reversible encephalopathy syndrome (PRES). The mechanism is cerebrovascular vasodilatation due to failure of autoregulation at such high blood pressures. Vascular permeability increases, and—together with comparative lack of sympathetic innervation in the posterior circulation that could constrict the arteries—may account for the proclivity for posteriorly located vasogenic cerebral edema. A third explanation is endothelial damage, altered vascular tone and permeability, and an inflammatory cytokine response leading to vasodilation. This mechanism is considered operative with chemotherapeutic drugs, calcineurin inhibitors, and sepsis. Usually a few generalized tonic-clonic seizures may accompany PRES. Single seizures are usually not treated with anti-epileptic drugs. A loading dose of phenytoin or levetiracetam may be used to cover the first days during recovery from the clinical manifestations of PRES.

A related disorder in pregnancy is eclampsia presenting with seizures, which is immediately concerning for the well-being of both the mother and the fetus. Management of seizures and hypertension is a key component of the management of eclampsia. Treatment is very different from that in other conditions. In patients with eclampsia, IV magnesium sulfate (titrating to a therapeutic serum level of magnesium, 2 to 3 mmol/L) is preferred, and the agent is more successful in seizure management than any other antiepileptic drug. Magnesium antagonizes and suppresses seizures mediated by the *N*-methyl-*D*-aspartate (NMDA) receptor. Moreover, although eclampsia comes late in pregnancy, there remains a concern that antiepileptic drugs or drugs to control status epilepticus may potentially cause harm to the fetus. These drugs are phenytoin, phenobarbital, valproate, and possibly the newer agent levetiracetam.

In most studies, recurrence of seizures after stroke is estimated at less than 10% in the first year, often combining ischemic with hemorrhagic stroke.[15,51] Status epilepticus from stroke was found in surprisingly high number of patients (19%)

in a large prospective series of patients with first-time strokes.[44] Early treatment, therefore, seems justified if seizures occur after ischemic or hemorrhagic stroke.

The need for antiepileptic drugs after aneurysmal subarachnoid hemorrhage remains unresolved and is only indicated if truly verified clinically or by EEG monitoring. Recurrence is more common in patients who have rebleed, have an associated hematoma, or are in a poor clinical grade. In these patients, prophylaxis with levetiracetam can be considered, but there remains insufficient evidence of its effect.[5,29]

Control of seizures can be achieved in each of these conditions, and outcome is generally good. Physicians have to be careful and more specific when they consider recurrent seizures a poor prognostic sign. The majority of patients may have a poor outcome from epilepsy-related causes. Mortality is most marked in the older age group and this may also reflect higher incidence of CNS neoplasms. Nonetheless, in a study of mortality in epilepsy, pneumonia was the cause of death and may reflect a terminal event rather than a cause of mortality.[28]

APPROACHING STATUS EPILEPTICUS

The outcome of nonconvulsive status epilepticus is more difficult to ascertain. The rhythmic EEG patterns need to be distinguished from triphasic waves, and nonconvulsive status epilepticus in the elderly is often overdiagnosed. Not surprisingly, a rapid clinical response to a single dose of intravenous benzodiazepine is the most important prognosticating factor in nonconvulsive status epilepticus. If the patient fails to improve after several doses of intravenous administration of benzodiazepine, or IV loading of phenytoin, valproate, or levetiracetam, nonconvulsive status epilepticus might be a manifestation of an injured brain rather than a treatable disorder.[20]

Outcome, however, is much different with convulsive status epilepticus. This will need to be distinguished from myoclonus status epilepticus. Even in the era of therapeutic hypothermia, generalized myoclonus status epilepticus as a result of anoxic-ischemic injury due to cardiac arrest remains associated with a very poor outcome (Chapter 3).

Variation in outcome in status epilepticus is considerable among reported clinical series. The major factors that determine outcome of status epilepticus are shown in Figure 4.1,[4,6,19,26] but no individual factor has been found to accurately predict outcome of status epilepticus. A recent study that summarized all successful cases found that the length of treatment of status epilepticus varied between roughly 1 and 15 months (average of 5 months). In all of these patients, multiple antiepileptic drugs—plus desperate measures such as electroshock treatment, and surgical extirpation of a potential focus—could still lead to a reasonable outcome.[21]

Some studies have suggested that more than one week's duration of status epilepticus may already indicate poor outcome, but other studies have found that this is an insufficient criterion. Encephalitis is often associated with a high

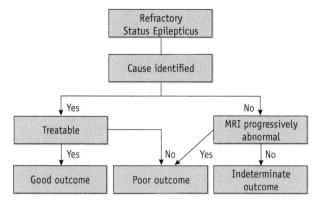

Figure 4.1 Algorithm for outcome of status epilepticus.

proportion of refractory status epilepticus, and patients who survive have a substantial risk of long-term seizures. Still outcome can be good in patients with comparatively normal MRI's outcome.[33–35] Conversely, poor outcome can be determined early if the underlying disorder is a terminal illness, such as recurrent glioblastoma or progressive metabolic disorders.

Another consideration is whether convulsive status epilepticus is associated with a CNS infection. This may be more prevalent in developing countries, where the cause of status epilepticus is far more commonly associated with neurocysticercosis, and in Asia, where it is associated with Japanese encephalitis. Tuberculosis and malaria are prevalent in sub-Saharan Africa, Southeast Asia, Latin America, and China.[3,13,48] In addition, particularly when it pertains to tuberculosis, there may be a coinfection with HIV. Some infections are associated with large epidemics such as dengue and influenza B.

There is one immediately pertinent practice issue: prediction of outcome in refractory status epilepticus. A comprehensive review of treatment for status epilepticus (refractory and super-refractory) in over 1,000 patients concluded that outcome was rarely mentioned (Table 4.1). It also became apparent that multiple therapies with changing doses are used, and therefore assessment of their individual effects was difficult to judge.[47]

Mortality in status epilepticus is most likely related to selection bias, treatment effects, and seizure type.[1,2,21,27,36,38,46,49] Unreliability of death certificates is also a major contributor; any prevalence study overrepresents people with more severe forms of status epilepticus. Most epilepsy cohorts also include myoclonus status epilepticus in the setting of anoxic-ischemic injury, presenting it erroneously as a potentially treatable disorder.

Patients with prolonged status epilepticus are at high risk of multiple medical complications; and outcome is largely determined by the ability to treat these medical complications and keep the patient in best medical condition to survive this neurocritical illness.[18,19,30] Patients treated with multiple doses of lorazepam and pentobarbital need to anticipate the potential for polyglycol toxicity causing

Table 4.1 **Published Literature on Treatment Outcomes in Status Epilepticus**

Therapy	*Number of Published Cases in Which Outcome Data Are Provided*
Midazolam	585
Pentobarbital/thiopental	192
Propofol	143
Topiramate	60
Emergency neurosurgery	36
Levetiracetam	35
Inhalational anesthetics	27
Immunotherapy	21
Ketamine	17
Ketogenic diet	14
Lacosamide	10
Hypothermia	9
ECT	8
Vagal nerve stimulation	4
Magnesium	3
CSF drainage	2

Source: Adapted from reference 47.

metabolic acidosis. Often metabolic acidosis is attributed to lactic acidosis, in turn attributed to ongoing seizures, and the real cause is missed (an osmolar gap will clinch the diagnosis). Bicarbonate infusions and continuous veno-venous hemofiltration (CCVH) may be needed in patients, but the condition is rare and more often found in patients with prior liver failure reducing the clearance of the toxic vehicle. Propofol is commonly used but not altogether safe and certainly not in high doses. Some studies have reported mortality due to propofol infusion syndrome.[22]

Every physician who takes care of a bedbound patient treated with anesthetic drugs has noted rapid skin breakdown, development of pleural effusions and infections, pulmonary emboli (despite prophylaxis), and even bacteremia and brief episodes of sepsis.[14] In addition, there is the potential for toxicity of antibiotics, particularly in vancomycin, that can damage kidney function significantly.

Patients may die during aggressive treatment or after withdrawal of support. The decision-making on withdrawal of care in these patients with refractory status epilepticus is not known in sufficient detail. It remains uncertain when physician and families decide that "enough is enough" after several unsuccessful attempts at weaning of anesthetic drugs. On the contrary, a persistently normal MRI in a patient treated for status epilepticus—not showing atrophy in the hippocampal areas or in the cortex—may still indicate a good chance of an acceptable outcome.

Morbidity in many of these patients continues to be very concerning, but the degree of disability has been less well studied. Very little is known of problems with day-to-day functioning, work challenges, and other major responsibilities. Survivors of status epilepticus due to prior neurologic injury (e.g., traumatic brain injury) have an increased risk of recurrence. Acute symptomatic status epilepticus has a greater than 40% chance of unprovoked seizures in the next decade. Recurrence rate of status epilepticus is low in patients without prior symptomatic status epilepticus.

By the Way

- It is difficult to define a point of no return in status epilepticus
- Rarely does a single drug finally treat refractory status epilepticus
- Status epilepticus is a treatable condition with possible good outcomes
- Status epilepticus requires long-term ICU care, and outcome may be determined by quality of care

---

Prognosis of Seizures and Status Epilepticus by the Numbers

- ~90% morbidity in refractory status epilepticus after 6 months
- ~50% mortality in refractory status epilepticus after 6 months
- ~40% of patients develop seizures after lobar hematoma
- ~10% of patients develop seizures after ischemic stroke
- ~10% of patients develop seizures after TBI

Putting It All Together

- Look for a structural lesion in recurrent seizures.
- Seizures due to posterior reversible encephalopathy syndrome are underappreciated and subside with blood pressure management
- Calcineurin neurotoxicity remains a common cause of seizures in organ transplant recipients, with no recurrence after replacement of the immunosuppressive drug
- Myoclonus status epilepticus as a result of anoxic-ischemic injury remains associated with a very poor outcome

- Outcome after refractory status epilepticus cannot be accurately assessed with repeatedly normal MRI
- Outcome after status epilepticus is largely determined by the ability to treat co-morbid medical complications

References

1. Bauer G, Trinka E. Nonconvulsive status epilepticus and coma. *Epilepsia* 2010;51:177–190.
2. Beghi E, Leone M, Solari A. Mortality in patients with a first unprovoked seizure. *Epilepsia* 2005;46:40–42.
3. Chen L, Zhou B, Li JM, et al. Clinical features of convulsive status epilepticus: a study of 220 cases in western China. *Eur J Neurol* 2009;16:444–449.
4. Claassen J, Lokin JK, Fitzsimmons BFM, Mendelsohn FA, Mayer SA. Predictors of functional disability and mortality after status epilepticus. *Neurology* 2002;58:139–142.
5. Connolly ES Jr, Rabinstein AA, Carhuapoma JR, et al. Guidelines for the management of aneurysmal subarachnoid hemorrhage: a guideline for healthcare professionals from the American Heart Association/American Stroke Association. *Stroke* 2012;43:1711–1737.
6. Cooper AD, Britton JW, Rabinstein AA. Functional and cognitive outcome in prolonged refractory status epilepticus. *Arch Neurol* 2009;66:1505–1509.
7. Costello DJ, Kilbride RD, Cole AJ. Cryptogenic new onset refractory status epilepticus (NORSE) in adults: infectious or not? *J Neurol Sci* 2009;277:26–31.
8. D'Ambrosio R, Maris DO, Grady MS, Winn HR, Janigro D. Impaired K(+) homeostasis and altered electrophysiological properties of post-traumatic hippocampal glia. *J Neurosci* 1999;19:8152–8162.
9. Delanty N, French JA, Labar DR, Pedley TA, Rowan AJ. Status epilepticus arising de novo in hospitalized patients: an analysis of 41 patients. *Seizure* 2001;10:116–119.
10. Drislane FW, Blum AS, Lopez MR, Schomer DL. Duration of refractory status epilepticus and outcome: loss of prognostic utility after several hours. *Epilepsia* 2009;50:1566–1571.
11. Drislane FW, Lopez MR, Blum AS, Schomer DL. Survivors and nonsurvivors of very prolonged status epilepticus. *Epilepsy Behav* 2011;22:342–345.
12. Foreman B, Hirsch LJ. Epilepsy emergencies: diagnosis and management. *Neurol Clin* 2012;30:11–41.
13. Forsgren L, Hauser WA, Olafsson E, et al. Mortality of epilepsy in developed countries: a review. *Epilepsia* 2005;46:18–27.
14. Fugate JE, Burns JD, Wijdicks EFM, et al. Prolonged high dose isoflurane for refractory status epilepticus: is it safe? *Anesth Analg* 2010;111:1520–1524.
15. Giroud M, Gras P, Fayolle H, et al. Early seizures after acute stroke: a study of 1,640 cases. *Epilepsia* 1994;35:959–964.
16. Graber KD, Prince DA. A critical period for prevention of posttraumatic neocortical hyperexcitability in rats. *Ann Neurol* 2004;55:860–870.
17. Hart YM, Sander JW, Johnson AL, Shorvon SD. National General Practice Study of Epilepsy: recurrence after a first seizure. *Lancet* 1990;336:1271–1274.
18. Hocker S, Britton JW, Mandrekar JN, Wijdicks EFM, Rabinstein AA. Predictors of outcome in refractory status epilepticus. *JAMA Neurol* 2013;70:72–77.
19. Holtkamp M, Othman J, Buchheim K, et al. A "malignant" variant of status epilepticus. *Arch Neurol* 2005;62:1428–1431.
20. Hopp JL, Sanchez A, Krumholz A, Hart G, Barry E. Nonconvulsive status epilepticus: value of a benzodiazepine trial for predicting outcomes. *Neurologist* 2011;17:325–329.
21. Hsieh CY, Sung PS, Tsai JJ, Huang CW. Terminating prolonged refractory status epilepticus using ketamine. *Clin Neuropharmacol* 2010;33:165–172.

22. Iyer VN, Hoel R, Rabinstein AA. Propofol infusion syndrome in patients with refractory status epilepticus: an 11-year clinical experience. *Crit Care Med* 2009;37:3024–3030.

23. Johnson N, Henry C, Fessler AJ, Dalmau J. Anti-NMDA receptor encephalitis causing prolonged nonconvulsive status epilepticus. *J Neurology* 2010;75:1480–1482.

24. Kaplan PW. No, some types of nonconvulsive status epilepticus cause little permanent neurologic sequelae (or: "the cure may be worse than the disease"). *Neurophysiol Clin* 2000;30:377–382.

25. Lee KR, Drury I, Vitarbo E, Hoff JT. Seizures induced by intracerebral injection of thrombin: a model of intracerebral hemorrhage. *J Neurosurg* 1997;87:73–78.

26. Legriel S, Azoulay E, Resche-Rigon M, et al. Functional outcome after convulsive status epilepticus. *Crit Care Med* 2010;38:2295–2303.

27. Legriel S, Mourvillier B, Bele N, et al. Outcomes in 140 critically ill patients with status epilepticus. *Intensive Care Med* 2008;34:476–480.

28. Lhatoo SD, Johnson AL, Goodridge DM, et al. Mortality in epilepsy in the first 11 to 14 years after diagnosis: multivariate analysis of a long-term, prospective, population-based cohort. *Ann Neurol* 2001;49:336–344.

29. Lindgren C, Nordh E, Naredi S, Olivecrona M. Frequency of non-convulsive seizures and non-convulsive status epilepticus in subarachnoid hemorrhage patients in need of controlled ventilation and sedation. *Neurocrit Care* 2012;17:367–373.

30. Logroscino G, Hesdorffer DC. Methodologic issues in studies of mortality following epilepsy: measures, types of studies, sources of cases, cohort effects, and competing risks. *Epilepsia* 2005;46:3–7.

31. Logroscino G, Hesdorffer DC, Cascino G, Annegers JF, Hauser WA. Short-term mortality after a first episode of status epilepticus. *Epilepsia* 1997;38:1344–1349.

32. Mirski MA, Williams MA, Hanley DF. Prolonged pentobarbital and phenobarbital coma for refractory generalized status epilepticus. *Crit Care Med* 1995;23:400–404.

33. Neligan A, Bell GS, Shorvon SD, Sander JW. Temporal trends in the mortality of people with epilepsy: a review. *Epilepsia* 2010;51:2241–2246.

34. Neligan A, Shorvon SD. Frequency and prognosis of convulsive status epilepticus of different causes: a systematic review. *Arch Neurol* 2010;67:931–940.

35. Neligan A, Shorvon SD. Prognostic factors, morbidity and mortality in tonic-clonic status epilepticus: a review. *Epilepsy Res* 2011;93:1–10.

36. Novy J, Logroscino G, Rossetti AO. Refractory status epilepticus: a prospective observational study. *Epilepsia* 2010;51:251–256.

37. Oddo M, Carrera E, Claassen J, Mayer SA, Hirsch LJ. Continuous electroencephalography in the medical intensive care unit. *Crit Care Med* 2009;37:2051–2056.

38. Power KN, Flaatten H, Gilhus NE, Engelsen BA. Propofol treatment in adult refractory status epilepticus: mortality risk and outcome. *Epilepsy Res* 2011;94:53–60.

39. Rossetti AO, Hurwitz S, Logroscino G, Bromfield EB. Prognosis of status epilepticus: role of aetiology, age, and consciousness impairment at presentation. *J Neurol Neurosurg Psychiatry* 2006;77:611–615.

40. Rossetti AO, Logroscino G, Bromfield EB. A clinical score for prognosis of status epilepticus in adults. *Neurology* 2006;66:1736–1738.

41. Rossetti AO, Logroscino G, Milligan TA, et al. Status Epilepticus Severity Score (STESS): a tool to orient early treatment strategy. *J Neurol* 2008;255:1561–1566.

42. Rossetti AO, Novy J, Ruffieux C, et al. Management and prognosis of status epilepticus according to hospital setting: a prospective study. *Swiss Med Wkly* 2009;139:719–723.

43. Rossetti AO, Oddo M. The neuro-ICU patient and electroencephalography paroxysms: if and when to treat. *Curr Opin Crit Care* 2010;16:105–109.

44. Rumbach L, Sablot D, Berger E, et al. Status epilepticus in stroke: report on a hospital-based stroke cohort. *Neurology* 2000;54:350–354.

45. Saz EU, Karapinar B, Ozcetin M, et al. Convulsive status epilepticus in children: etiology, treatment protocol and outcome. *Seizure* 2011;20:115–118.

46. Shackleton DP, Westendorp RG, Kasteleijn-Nolst Trenité DG, de Craen AJ, Vandenbroucke JP. Survival of patients with epilepsy: an estimate of the mortality risk. *Epilepsia* 2002;43:445–450.
47. Shorvon S, Ferlisi M. The treatment of super-refractory status epilepticus: a critical review of available therapies and a clinical treatment protocol. *Brain* 2011;134:2802–2818.
48. Singhi P. Infectious causes of seizures and epilepsy in the developing world. *Dev Med Child Neurol* 2011;53:600–609.
49. Sperling MR, Feldman H, Kinman J, Liporace JD, O'Connor MJ. Seizure control and mortality in epilepsy. *Ann Neurol* 1999;46:45–50.
50. Standley K, Abdulmassih R, Benbadis S. Good outcome is possible after months of refractory convulsive status epilepticus: lesson learned. *Epilepsia* 2012;53:e17–e20.
51. Varelas PN. *Seizures in Critical Care: A Guide to Diagnosis and Management* 2nd ed. New York, Humana Press, 2010.

5

Prognostication After CNS Infections

Central nervous system (CNS) infections are typically isolated events caused by commensal or community-acquired organisms, but may be epidemic. Emerging infections and pandemics have also been associated with CNS infections—most notable are West Nile virus (WNV). Other infections, such as severe acute respiratory syndrome (SARS) or influenza A (H1N1), do not directly infect CNS but secondarily, through the effects of sepsis and severe hypoxemia, damage the brain. Most hospitals in the developed world will admit patients with acute bacterial meningitis from *Streptococcus pneumoniae* or *Neisseria meningitidis*. In developing (often tropical) countries, the incidence of bacterial meningitis is more than five times higher than in the developed world outcome is almost 10 times worse, particularly in children.[1]

Encephalitis is usually due to a herpes simplex virus or a nondistinct virus but now probably more commonly due to an autoimmune process. Some patients die as a result of encephalitis or meningitis, a substantial proportion is disabled and not the same after this event, and even in recovered patients it is not uncommon for them to seek assistance. The outcome is different when young adults and children are compared with the elderly, but the age cutoff is likely already at the second or third decade, suggesting that only the very young are able to sustain such an onslaught to the central nervous system.

In many types of encephalitis, no specific treatment exists, and outcome is largely determined by the degree of supportive care, control of seizures and occasionally control of increased intracranial pressure. Many CNS infections can be overcome, with subsequent recovery of the patient. Some encephalitides are so rapidly severe in presentation that patients may end up in a minimally conscious state or a persistent vegetative state.

Several questions remain before clinicians can decide on outcome: What specific treatments are available, and how do we best aggressively approach a CNS infection in order to improve outcome? Which CNS infections are neurosurgical emergencies? How is the outcome different in immunocompromised patients? This chapter addresses the most common CNS infections and expected for outcome.

Principles

There are some very specific pieces of information required when assessing outcome of CNS infection. A first core principle is that outcome of any type of brain infection is likely determined by the time it took to recognize it in the first place[4], and by the time it took to treat with adequate and appropriate doses of antimicrobial medication.[20,35,38–41] More than with any other acute brain injury, misjudgments are frequently made in clinical assessment and management of CNS infections. This is particularly true in immunocompromised patients, where the clinical presentation of a CNS infection is nonspecific and may simply lack the conventional clinical pointers.

When acute bacterial meningitis is suspected, a well-accepted diagnostic and therapeutic pathway is to first rapidly obtain blood cultures, proceed with IV antibiotics and IV antivirals, consider IV corticosteroids, and order a CT scan to exclude mass occupying effect before proceeding with a lumbar puncture. Thus, in the evaluation of the patient, outcome can get unexpectedly worse if the decision is made to do a lumbar puncture before a CT scan in a patient who has already developed severe cerebral edema, and in a patient with an epidural empyema and mass effect, both conditions that are clinically indistinguishable from any fulminant bacterial infection.

An important determinant is whether the patient with bacterial meningitis has been treated with corticosteroids, which in several studies have changed outcome in a significant manner.[3,8,36,37] High-dose dexamethasone is beneficial in adults and particularly in children with *Haemophilus influenzae* meningitis (rare now). Its benefit is inconclusive in childhood pneumococcal meningitis, but it has been proven effective in adult pneumococcal meningitis. Early treatment, if available, confers a significant benefit not only in survival but also morbidity. There is a sense in the infectious medical community that treating a patient with fulminant meningitis with dexamethasone is not an option—it is an obligation.

Outcome is also determined by the aggressiveness of care. Clearly, it remains important to know whether the physician is willing to aggressively treat early and late complications. Brain edema can in some instances be effectively treated with osmotic diuretics and additional high-dose IV corticosteroids, and acute obstructive hydrocephalus should be treated with placement of a ventriculostomy. If CT or MRI show the presence of ventricular empyema or ventriculitis, they may be treated with intrathecal antibiotics after access is obtained.

In some patients meningitis is complicated by thrombophlebitis. When local (close to the mastoiditis) it requires immediate otolaryngeal expertise and surgery. Although uncertain extensive thrombophlebitis could potentially benefit from anticoagulation. None of these interventions have proven to be effective, but no action of this sort will certainly result in a poor outcome.[28] Some infections of the CNS are associated with sepsis, and the ability to treat sepsis—often associated with multiorgan failure—also can influence outcome. The most important example is the development of septicemia in *Neisseria* meningitis. In a matter of hours (often early in disease presentation), an inflammation is built up into diffuse intravascular coagulation, and widespread purpura. Shock is often refractory with cardiovascular collapse. Therefore, patients with a CNS infection may succumb as a direct consequence of a secondary systemic infection. Septic shock was seen in nearly 30% of patients with severe bacterial meningitis studied in a recent prospective clinical trial.[24]

In encephalitis, the main distinguishing factor is whether the patient has encephalitis that can potentially be treated with antiviral medication. Treatment is immediately needed in herpes zoster or herpes simplex encephalitis.[23] Many of the seasonal arbovirus-associated encephalitides do not have a specific treatment, and outcome in the more severely affected patients is entirely dependent on intensive care support. What also has become apparent over several years is that the category "viral encephalitis" may have included autoimmune encephalitis, and recognition of this subset may lead to a different outcome if appropriate therapies—a combination of corticosteroids and rituximab—are provided. In some patients with autoimmune encephalitis, an aggressive search for a trigger (e.g., a microscopic ovarian teratoma) may pay off.[7] Ovariectomy may lead to a marked improvement of clinical manifestations in these patients—often young, previously healthy females (see volume *Handling Difficult Situations*).

Finally, several infections are neurosurgical emergencies. This includes any cranial or spinal epidural empyema, cerebral abscesses, and ventriculitis. Each of these disorders can be treated effectively if recognized, washed out or drained, and treated with multiple antibiotics immediately after admission.

A second core principle is that recovery from a recent CNS infection—no matter what the cause—takes time and is protracted. If early withdrawal of care is proposed in a patient who remains comatose several days after antibiotic or antiviral treatment, outcome obviously will be worse. Physicians should resist de-escalation of care if the patient has "plateaued" for several weeks and, in particular, if there is no other reason that makes improvement unlikely. However, major complications may recur, and these are cerebral infarcts, cerebral phlebitis,[32] or cerebral edema not responding to osmotic diuretics and high-dose corticosteroids.

A third core principle is that CNS infections in immunocompromised patients not only have different etiologies but also very different outcomes. *Listeria meningitis* is more common in the elderly with prior malignancies and after an organ transplant.[25] Patients with human immunodeficiency virus (HIV) infection have a considerable risk of developing toxoplasmic encephalitis, cytomegalovirus encephalitis, cryptococcal meningitis, and other rarely seen parasitic and fungal infections. Antiretroviral therapy after such infections emerge has important consequences, with less recurrences and improved survival. Central nervous system tuberculosis with associated miliary lesions and co-infection with HIV all reduce the chances of recovery. Insurmountable barriers to treatment may play a large role, and delay in presentation is common.

Immunocompromised patients are also at some risk of infection, with the JC virus causing progressive multifocal leukoencephalopathy. This neurodegenerative disease remains associated with poor outcome and rapid demise (months) except in patients with low JC virus load in cerebrospinal fluid (CSF) and high CD4 counts at the time of diagnosis. Most commonly, the severity of manifestations (rapidly developing brainstem involvement and dementia) often determines the outcome, rather than laboratory criteria or response of viral load to cidofovir.[6]

In Practice

Some generalizations in outcome assessment in common CNS infections may apply and guidance is shown in Figure 5.1. Clearly further differentiation is needed, and the most commonly encountered infections need more detailed discussion.

Bacterial CNS infections usually result in a significant injury to the brain. More to the point, mortality in most published clinical series is approximately 10% to 15%. In survivors of bacterial meningitis, the length of stay in the ICU and later the hospital ward usually ranges from one to three weeks.

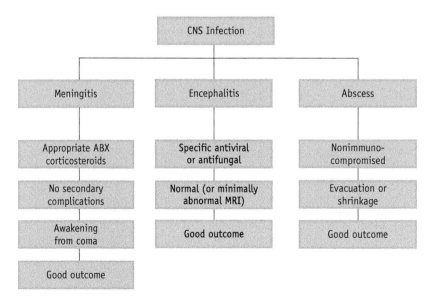

Figure 5.1 Outcome in meningitis, encephalitis, and cerebral abscess. ABX: antibiotics; MRI: magnetic resonance imaging.

Table 5.1 **Prognostic Factors in Adults with CNS Infections**

• Ventriculomegaly
• Extensive thrombophlebitis
• Cerebral edema
• Multiple septic infarctions
• Diffuse MRI abnormalities (including hippocampi)
• Any major systemic illness including multiorgan failure and shock

In acute bacterial meningitis, the cortex is often involved, and most patients have a meningoencephalitis. Complications that may occur include seizures, acute hydrocephalus, and septic cerebral infarctions, which all determine the degree of morbidity. Multiorgan failure and septic shock may be the first presentation in a patient with bacterial meningitis. The most important factor associated with poor outcome in bacterial meningitis is a systemic illness that manifests itself by tachycardia, hypotension, thrombocytopenia and positive blood cultures.[5,12,13,15,33] Etiology matters, and the odds of unfavorable outcome are six times higher in patients infected with *S. pneumoniae* than in patients infected with *N. meningitidis*. Presence of CT scan abnormalities that show ventriculomegaly is a poor prognosticator; the same applies to diffuse brain edema. Most studies have found that delay in onset of treatment is associated with adverse clinical outcome (Table 5.1).[4]

The age of the patient is also an important prognosticating factor. An immature immune status results in more severe infections. Several important prognosticating factors have been identified in neonates and young children (Table 5.2).[2,26,29,30]. In children, for some inexplicable reason, male gender was also found to be an

Table 5.2 **Prognostic Factors in Children with CNS Infections**

• Onset >48 h
• Coma
• Seizures
• Shock
• Severe respiratory distress syndrome
• Prolonged fever (>7 days)
• Low peripheral WBC count
• Low CSF WBC count, glucose or protein
• *S. pneumonia* as causative pathogen

WBC = white blood cell count; CSF = cerebrospinal fluid.
Source: Data from references 9, 11, 14, 16, 18, and 21.

important factor. Neurologic sequelae (e.g., hearing loss),[22] focal neurologic findings (e.g., hemiparesis or aphasia), and cognitive impairment may occur in up to one-third of the patients, and again more frequently with pneumococcal meningitis rather than meningococcal meningitis.

Responsiveness to antibiotic therapy may be influenced by several factors, predominantly the penetration into the brain and whether adequate bacterial activity in CSF can be achieved where it is needed. In a patient who is not improving, a repeat CSF may not document sterility, in which case intraventricular vancomycin could be administered. Susceptibility testing may direct which antibiotics to use. For many years, *S. pneumoniae* strains have been only intermediately susceptible to penicillin and require either cefotaxime or ceftriaxone in a high dose. Meningitis is also treated with vancomycin if high-level resistance to β-lactam antibiotics is suspected.

It has remained unclear whether hypothermia improves outcome in bacterial meningitis. A recent clinical trial prematurely ended when outcome in hypothermia-treated patients was worse. However, outcome in this study was very poor, suggesting either moribund patients at entry or less aggressive management in major aspects of care.[24]

Brain abscesses may be the result of metastatic spread from an endocarditis or from hematogenous spread of fungi. The source needs to be identified and may be from oral infections (these may not be visually apparent and would need an orthopantomogram), paranasal sinuses, otitis media, or from penetrating trauma. *Streptococcus milleri* is most common in abscesses associated with paranasal sinusitis. Otogenic abscesses are commonly caused by *Proteus* anaerobes, *Streptococcus* species, Enterobacteriaceae, or *Pseudomonas aeruginosa*.

The outcome of a single brain abscess is dependent on whether the patient is a good surgical candidate and most patients with an isolated lesion are. The threshold for a neurosurgical approach should also be low if the abscess is superficially located or in the cerebellum. Antimicrobial therapy seems more appropriate in patients with deep-seated abscesses or multilocular abscesses and in immunosuppressed patients with disseminated microabscesses caused by toxoplasmosis or aspergillosis.

Enlargement of the abscess with gradual clinical deterioration is an absolute indication for stereotactic aspiration or extirpation. Outcome seems correlated with location of lesion (deep-seated), progression to coma before intervention, and, particularly, ventricular rupture.

Empiric therapy of a surgically inaccessible lesion in a nonimmunocompromised patient is metronidazole, vancomycin, and a third- or fourth-generation cephalosporin. Meropenem has been added if *P. aeruginosa* is suspected, but this is usually avoided due to high risk of seizures in any patient with an abscess (cefepime or ceftazidime are better options). Corticosteroids may reduce antibiotic penetration and are usually only administered before and after neurosurgical extirpation.

One of the most concerning bacterial infections to the brain are patients with an epidural or subdural empyema. The infection may progress slowly initially and usually originates from a chronic sinusitis or recent sinus surgery. Frontal or periorbital swelling are useful clinical clues, but the disorder is notoriously difficult to recognize clinically, with fever or no fever, focal findings or no focal findings, seizures or no seizures. Unrelenting headache may be the only clinical sign in a patient with a prior sinusitis. CT scan may be diagnostic only if contrast is administered that shows the inflamed convex-shaped ring close to the bone. Here again, early recognition and aggressive triple antibiotic or antifungal treatment can result in control. Invasive mucormycosis may even be successfully treated in the majority of the cases, although this type of sinusitis remains associated with mortality in about a third of patients. Outcome of a subdural or epidural empyema is entirely determined by the presence of coma before surgery, and mortality is then high (up to 80%). Surviving patients often have a residual hemiparesis and a seizure disorder.

Outcome of encephalitis with cerebral edema remains poor. It is also determined largely by whether the patient has an encephalitis that can be treated with specific antimicrobial drugs or whether status epilepticus emerges.[17,19,33] Many variables have been identified and include age, duration of disease, and level of consciousness. Patients who are younger than 30 years of age and remain largely alert have a much higher chance of returning to normal life than patients who are older and have altered consciousness.

The time to start treatment with IV acyclovir also determines outcome and mortality, and early treatment is obviously warranted. Outcome is better if patients are treated within 4 days. Delay of treatment in some patients is understandable, because in many patients with herpes simplex encephalitis, acute confusion and febrile episodes are not appreciated as severe until the patient develops a seizure or develops recognizable clinical findings. Nevertheless, less than 20% of patients, despite treatment with IV acyclovir, have a completely normal outcome. Moderate to severe cognitive impairments leading to inability to hold a job[10,31] were found in the overwhelming majority of patients.[31] Mortality remains quite high and may reach 50%, mostly as a result of withdrawal of support in the elderly and particularly if the patient remains comatose. More effective antiviral regimens would be welcomed.

Some encephalitides have a poor outcome, and no treatment is effective. This includes rabies encephalitis, many of the fungal infections, and more recently West Nile virus (WNV) encephalitis. West Nile virus encephalitis has been a major infection in the summer months after a major sweep in the US from east to west from 1999 to 2009 (there has been recent flare ups in Texas). Its management is supportive. Many patients with fever or meningitis recover fully, but the more neuroinvasive form can cause a flaccid paralysis and marked changes in basal ganglia, thalami, and brainstem. Generally there is a 20% mortality rate for WNV encephalitis and 10%–15% mortality for patients with acute WNV myelitis, with mortality higher in the elderly patient. If a patient is comatose from WNV encephalitis, the chance of recovery without any major neurologic deficit is low.[27] However, some patients are only mildly "encephalopathic" and can make a full recovery. Parkinsonism is also a common residual feature and is explained by the presence of the virus in the substantia nigra and basal ganglia. Patients with a WNV myelopathy only partially improve, with many suffering persistent residual limb weakness. Most unfortunately, patients who require mechanical ventilation are not commonly weaned off the ventilator and require permanent tracheostomy and mechanical ventilation.[27] Human vaccines of WNV are not yet available. Outcome categorized by infectious agent is shown in Table 5.3.

The most difficult situation arises in a patient who is immunocompromised. This may be a patient after organ transplantation or a patient on corticosteroids for vasculitic or autoimmune syndromes and certain neurologic disorders such as myasthenia gravis. Any immunocompromised patient presenting with a fulminant meningitis and "yeast" in CSF most likely has a *Cryptococcus neoformans* infection. Clinical symptoms are very often initally absent, subtle, or fluctuating in severity. Persistent headache may be the only symptom that points to the infection. A CSF examination can yield high opening pressures, normal cell count, and findings expected in fungal meningitis, such as lymphocytic pleocytosis and reduced glucose. In 95% of patients, the diagnosis can be confirmed by CSF culture and serologic detection of CSF cryptococcal antigen (titers of 1:32 or more). Serum cryptococcal antigen can be found in virtually all cases.

There are other unique features of CNS infection in patients who are organ transplant recipients. Systemic viral infections may emerge after transplantation but most often are expected 1 to 6 months after grafting. A systemic viremia is often present in patients with CNS involvement, and some viral infections

Table 5.3 **Outcome in Encephalitides**

Encephalitis	Outcome	Predictors for Poor Outcome
Herpes Simplex	Intermediate	Time to Rx with acyclovir
Tick-borne	Poor	Coma
Toxoplasmic	Intermediate	HIV
Cryptococcus	Poor	Obstructive hydrocephalus and increased ICP
Progressive multifocal leukoencephalopathy	Poor	High JC virus load in CSF
Fungal	Good/intermediate	Relapse
Tuberculosis	Poor	Miliary

Rx = treatment; ICP = intracranial pressure; JC = John Cunningham; CSF = cerebrospinal fluid; HIV = Human immunodeficiency virus.

in immunocompromised patients can cause fulminant and lethal disseminated infections. Human herpesvirus 6 (HHV-6) infection can be transmitted through the graft and cause a life-threatening infection, and may appear within the first postoperative month. There are clinical similarities with immunosuppression neurotoxicity, but MRI shows multiple nonenhancing lesions in gray matter without any predilection. Most patients with HHV-6 encephalitis present similar to that of limbic encephalitis.

Immunocompromised transplant recipients are also particularly susceptible to *L. monocytogenes* and *Nocardia asteroïdes*. Immunocompromised patients with ring-like and hemorrhagic parenchymal lesions may have nocardial abscesses. The most frequent clinical presentation of listeriosis is acute meningitis with fever and headache. Clinical signs with dysarthria and dysphagia may be due to a predilection of *Listeria* for the brain stem.

By the Way

- Corticosteroids halves mortality rate in fulminant meningitis
- Mortality in septic sagittal sinus thrombosis is high
- 1 in 10 patients with *Neisseria* meningitis develops septicemia
- 1 in 3 patients with severe meningitis develop sepsis
- Mortality after brain abscess has declined due to early recognition

---

CNS infection By the Numbers

- ~100% mortality in rabies encephalitis
- ~80% mortality of CNS infections caused by fungal infections
- ~70% mortality with *Staphylococcus aureus* meningitis
- ~30% mortality with *Pneumococcal* meningitis
- ~10% mortality with *Neisseria* meningitis

Putting It All Together

- Recognition of CNS infections remains a challenge for most physicians
- Early aggressive treatment in bacterial meningitis is key
- Effective treatment of complications could impact on outcome in CNS infections
- There is often a major delay in treating herpes simplex virus encephalitis
- Seasonal encephalitis causes significant morbidity
- Given the poor prognosis of CNS infections in immunosuppressed patients, it is unclear whether recognition and early treatment improves outcome

References

1. Akpede GO, Akuhwa RT, Ogiji EO, Ambe JP. Risk factors for an adverse outcome in bacterial meningitis in the tropics: a reappraisal with focus on the significance and risk of seizures. *Ann Trop Paediatr* 1999;19:151–159.
2. Anderson V, Anderson P, Grimwood K, Nolan T. Cognitive and executive function 12 years after childhood bacterial meningitis: effect of acute neurologic complications and age of onset. *J Pediatr Psychol* 2004;29:67–81.
3. Annane D, Sébille V, Charpentier C, et al. Effect of treatment with low doses of hydrocortisone and fludrocortisone on mortality in patients with septic shock. *JAMA* 2002;288:862–871.
4. Aronin SI, Peduzzi P, Quagliarello VJ. Community-acquired bacterial meningitis: risk stratification for adverse clinical outcome and effect of antibiotic timing. *Ann Intern Med* 1998;129:862–869.
5. Auburtin M, Porcher R, Bruneel F, et al. Pneumococcal meningitis in the intensive care unit: prognostic factors of clinical outcome in a series of 80 cases. *Am J Respir Crit Care Med* 2002;165:713–717.
6. Berenguer J, Miralles P, Arrizabalaga J, et al. Clinical course and prognostic factors of progressive multifocal leukoencephalopathy in patients treated with highly active antiretroviral therapy. *Clin Infect Dis* 2003;36:1047–1052.
7. Dalmau J, Lancaster E, Martinez-Hernandez E, Rosenfeld MR, Balice-Gordon R. Clinical experience and laboratory investigations in patients with anti-NMDAR encephalitis. *Lancet Neurol* 2011;10:63–74.
8. de Gans J, van de Beek D; European Dexamethasone in Adulthood Bacterial Meningitis Study Investigators. Dexamethasone in adults with bacterial meningitis. *N Engl J Med* 2002;347:1549–1556.
9. de Jonge RC, van Furth AM, Wassenaar M, Gemke RJ, Terwee CB. Predicting sequelae and death after bacterial meningitis in childhood: a systematic review of prognostic studies. *BMC Infect Dis* 2010;10:232.
10. Elbers JM, Bitnun A, Richardson SE, et al. A 12-year prospective study of childhood herpes simplex encephalitis: is there a broader spectrum of disease? *Pediatrics* 2007;119:e399–e407.
11. Fakhir S, Ahmad SH, Ahmad P. Prognostic factors influencing mortality in meningococcal meningitis. *Ann Trop Paediatr* 1992;12:149–154.
12. Fitch MT, van de Beek D. Emergency diagnosis and treatment of adult meningitis. *Lancet Infect Dis* 2007;7:191–200.
13. Flores-Cordero JM, Amaya-Villar R, Rincón-Ferrari MD, et al. Acute community-acquired bacterial meningitis in adults admitted to the intensive care unit: clinical manifestations, management and prognostic factors. *Intensive Care Med* 2003;29:1967–1973.

14. Fowler A, Stödberg T, Eriksson M, Wickström R. Childhood encephalitis in Sweden: etiology, clinical presentation and outcome. *Eur J Paediatr Neurol* 2008;12:484–490.
15. Granerod J, Ambrose HE, Davies NW, et al. Causes of encephalitis and differences in their clinical presentations in England: a multicentre, population-based prospective study. *Lancet Infect Dis* 2010;10:835–844.
16. Grimwood K, Nolan TM, Bond L, Anderson VA, Catroppa C, Keir EH. Risk factors for adverse outcomes of bacterial meningitis. *J Paediatr Child Health* 1996;32:457–462.
17. Halperin JJ. *Encephalitis: Diagnosis and Management.* New York, Informa Healthcare, 2008.
18. Kaaresen PI, Flaegstad T. Prognostic factors in childhood bacterial meningitis. *Acta Paediatr* 1995;84:873–878.
19. Kennedy PG. Viral encephalitis. *J Neurol* 2005;252:268–272.
20. Klein M, Pfister HW, Leib SL, Koedel U. Therapy of community-acquired acute bacterial meningitis: the clock is running. *Expert Opin Pharmacother* 2009;10:2609–2623.
21. Kornelisse RF, Westerbeek CM, Spoor AB, et al. Pneumococcal meningitis in children: prognostic indicators and outcome. *Clin Infect Dis* 1995;21:1390–1397.
22. Kutz JW, Simon LM, Chennupati SK, Giannoni CM, Manolidis S. Clinical predictors for hearing loss in children with bacterial meningitis. *Arch Otolaryngol Head Neck Surg* 2006;132:941–945.
23. McGrath N, Anderson NE, Croxson MC, Powell KF. Herpes simplex encephalitis treated with acyclovir: diagnosis and long term outcome. *J Neurol Neurosurg Psychiatry* 1997;63:321–326.
24. Mourvillier B, Tuback F, van de Beek D, et al. Induced hypothermia in severe bacterial meningitis: a randomized clinical trial. *JAMA* 2013;310:2174–2183.
25. Mylonakis E, Hohmann EL, Calderwood SB. Central nervous system infection with *Listeria monocytogenes*: 33 years' experience at a general hospital and review of 776 episodes from the literature. *Medicine* 1998;77:313–336.
26. Oostenbrink R, Maas M, Moons KG, Moll HA. Sequelae after bacterial meningitis in childhood. *Scand J Infect Dis* 2002;34:379–382.
27. Petersen LR, Brault AC, Nasci RS. West nile virus: review of the literature. *JAMA* 2013;310:308–315.
28. Pfister HW, Feiden W, Einhäupl KM. Spectrum of complications during bacterial meningitis in adults: results of a prospective clinical study. *Arch Neurol* 1993;50:575–581.
29. Pomeroy SL, Holmes SJ, Dodge PR, Feigin RD. Seizures and other neurologic sequelae of bacterial meningitis in children. *N Engl J Med* 1990;323:1651–1657.
30. Radcliffe RH. Review of the NICE guidance on bacterial meningitis and meningococcal septicaemia. *Arch Dis Child Educ Pract Ed* 2011;96:234–237.
31. Raschilas F, Wolff M, Delatour F, et al. Outcome of and prognostic factors for herpes simplex encephalitis in adult patients: results of a multicenter study. *Clin Infect Dis* 2002;35:254–260.
32. Rubin M, Wijdicks EFM. Fulminant streptococcal meningoencephalitis. *JAMA Neurol* 2013;70:515.
33. Thakur KT, Motta M, Asemota AO, et al. Predictors of outcome in acute encephalitis. *Neurology* 2013;81:783–800.
34. Thompson C, Kneen R, Riordan A, Kelly D, Pollard AJ. Encephalitis in children. *Arch Dis Child* 2012;97:150–161.
35. van de Beek D, de Gans J, Tunkel AR, Wijdicks EFM. Community-acquired bacterial meningitis in adults. *N Engl J Med* 2006;354:44–53.
36. Weisfelt M, Hoogman M, van de Beek D, et al. Dexamethasone and long-term outcome in adults with bacterial meningitis. *Ann Neurol* 2006;60:456–468.
37. Weisfelt M, van de Beek D, Spanjaard L, Reitsma JB, de Gans J. Clinical features, complications, and outcome in adults with pneumococcal meningitis: a prospective case series. *Lancet Neurol* 2006;5:123–129.
38. Whitley RJ, Alford CA, Hirsch MS, et al. Vidarabine versus acyclovir therapy in herpes simplex encephalitis. *N Engl J Med* 1986;314:144–149.

39. Whitley RJ. Herpes simplex encephalitis: adolescents and adults. *Antiviral Res* 2006;71: 141–148.

40. Whitley RJ, Soong SJ, Dolin R, et al. Adenine arabinoside therapy of biopsy-proved herpes simplex encephalitis: National Institute of Allergy and Infectious Diseases collaborative antiviral study. *N Engl J Med* 1977;297:289–294.

41. Whitley RJ, Soong SJ, Hirsch MS, et al. Herpes simplex encephalitis: vidarabine therapy and diagnostic problems. *N Engl J Med* 1981;304:313–318.

6

Prognostication After Acute Neuromuscular Disorders

For many decades, treatment of acute severe neuromuscular disease emphasized supportive care, and the degree to which it could be provided determined outcome. Now, with more therapeutic options directed at specific targets together with much improved respiratory support—and needless to say neurocritical care— the outcome for many of these disorders has changed.

Acute neuromuscular disorders may rapidly cause major paralysis, and the patient and the patient's family often are keen to hear the outcome. Prediction of outcome comes up when the patient has reached a presumable nadir and improvement seems far away. Furthermore, the psychological impact of realizing there potentially may be permanent disability is substantial. Prognosis in the setting of an acute neuromuscular disorder is also often discussed after the patient has been mechanically ventilated and following unsuccessful weaning attempts.

In neurology practices, acute or subacute neuromuscular diseases most commonly seen are: Guillain-Barré syndrome (GBS), acute myasthenia gravis, and amyotrophic lateral sclerosis (ALS). Rarely one may encounter acute myopathy syndromes, acute vasculitis neuropathies, or even tick paralysis. In some patients who have survived a critical illness—often associated with a severe sepsis syndrome—an acute neuromuscular disorder may be partly a consequence of inflammatory response to critical illness or a consequence of drugs to treat critical illness, such as intravenous corticosteroids combined with neuromuscular junction blockers. In developing countries, tetanus and botulism remain prevalent, but a rarity in other parts of the world.

Knowledge of prognosis in acute neuromuscular disorders serves an important purpose. One could reasonably define a good outcome as a patient (1) who returns to walking with or without support[51]; (2) who has no need for ventilatory support, and whose tracheostomy has been removed; (3) whose swallowing mechanism has recovered; (4) who has the ability to read with or without corrective measures[7]; (5) who has no fatigue, signs of depression, or major inactivity[32]; and (6) who has no major bladder disturbances.[28] Each of these criteria will in some way define the quality of life in a patient acutely stricken by this disorder. So important questions are as follows: Who is going to recover fully and why? What is the level of rehabilitation intensity? How do we measure disability in these disorders? What can we do to improve quality of life if no improvement or even further progression is expected? This chapter provides some insight.

Principles

One of the first core principles is that the level of ICU care may change outcome of neuromuscular disorders.[26,29] This may not seem so obvious, but failure to adequately manage medical complications of mechanical ventilation (i.e., ventilator-associated pneumonia or ventilator-associated gastrointestinal bleeding) may jeopardize the patient's outcome, despite a stable or even improving neurologic deficit. Time on the ventilator is an important prognosticator in any acute neuromuscular disorder for the simple reason that it increases the risk of medical complications.[17,45,46] Dysphagia and respiratory dysfunction commonly go together in acute neuromuscular disorders and may lead to pooling secretions and aspiration. One can imagine that the elderly patient with aspiration due to marked oropharyngeal dysfunction who is subsequently intubated and mechanically ventilated may need not only aggressive antibiotic coverage but also many other supportive measures. Ventilator-associated pneumonia prolongs time on the ventilator, complicates weaning efforts, and increases the chance of tracheostomy and introduces additional risks such as dislodgment and bleeding at the site.

A second core principle is that the degree of weakness at first presentation may predict recovery time. It is useful to adequately categorize weakness. Weakness is universally determined by the Medical Research Council (MRC) metric, and some modification has been suggested for use in these patients.[52] It is useful to stick to six key muscle groups in the extremities (Table 6.1). Besides limb weakness, this

Table 6.1 **Medical Research Council (MRC) Sum Score**

0 No visible contraction
1 Visible contraction without movement of the limb
2 Active movement of the limb, but not against gravity
3 Active movement against gravity over (almost) the full range
4 Active movement against gravity and resistance
5 Normal power

The MRC score of an individual muscle group ranges from 0 to 5. Sum of MRC scores of six bilateral muscle groups, includes shoulder abductors, elbow flexors, wrist extensors, hip flexors, knee extensors, and foot dorsiflexors, ranging from 60 (normal) to 0 (quadriplegic).

Table 6.2 **GBS Disability Score**

0 A healthy state
1 Minor symptoms and capable of running
2 Able to walk 10 m or more without assistance but unable to run
3 Able to walk 10 m across an open space with help
4 Bedridden or chair bound
5 Requiring assisted ventilation for at least part of the day

includes ocular, faciopharyngeal and truncal weakness. Impairment may cause inability to sit up from a lying position, ptosis, double vision, and inability to chew or swallow or to speak clearly. Acute neuromuscular disorders will have certain similarities but also differences and patterns that fit best with that disorder. Quantitative scales should have a number of specific items to be potentially helpful. Validated quantitative scales have been developed for GBS, myasthenia gravis and ALS. They are shown in Tables 6.2 to 6.4.[4,5]

Table 6.3 **The Quantitative Myasthenia Gravis Score**

Test Item	None	Mild	Moderate	Severe
Grade	0	1	2	3
Ptosis (upward gaze), sec	60	11–59	1–10	Spontaneous
Diplopia (lateral gaze), R or L, s	60	11–59	1–10	Spontaneous
Eyelid closure	Normal	Complete, some resistance	Complete, no resistance	Incomplete
Dysarthria with counting 1–50	None at # 50	Dysarthria at # 30–49	Dysarthria at # 10–29	Dysarthria at # 9
Swallowing 1/2 cup	Normal	Mild cough, throat clearing	Severe cough/ choking	Unable
Vital capacity, % predicted	≥80%	65–79%	50–64%	<50%
Right arm held out-stretched at 90°, s	240	90–239	10–89	0–9
Left arm held out-stretched at 90°, s	240	90–239	10–89	0–9
Right hand grip, kgW, man/woman	≥45/≥30	15–44/10–29	5–14/5–9	0–4/0–4
Left hand grip, kgW, man/woman	≥35/≥25	15–34/10–24	5–14/5–9	0–4/0–4

(continued)

Table 6.3 **Continued**

Test Item	None	Mild	Moderate	Severe
Head lift 45° supine, sec	120	30–119	1–29	0
Right leg held outstretched at 45° supine, sec	100	31–99	1–30	0
Left leg outstretched at 45° supine, sec	100	31–99	1–30	0

Table 6.4 **The Amyotrophic Lateral Sclerosis Functional Rating Scale (ALSFRS)**

Measure	Finding	Points
Speech	Normal	4
	Detectable speech disturbance	3
	Intelligible with repeating	2
	Speech combined with nonvocal communications	1
	Loss of useful speech	0
Salivation	Normal	4
	Slight but definite excess of saliva in mouth; may have nighttime drooling	3
	Moderately excessive saliva; may have minimal drooling	2
	Marked excess of saliva with some drooling	1
	Marked drooling; requires constant tissue or handkerchief	0
Swallowing	Normal	4
	Early eating problems; occasional choking	3
	Dietary consistency changes	2
	Needs supplemental tube feedings	1
	Nothing by mouth (NPO); exclusively parenteral or enteral feeding	0
Handwriting	Normal	4
	Slow or sloppy; all words are legible	3
	Not all words are legible	2
	Able to grasp pen but unable to write	1
	Unable to grip pen	0
Cutting food and handling utensils	No gastrostomy/normal	4

(continued)

Table 6.4 **Continued**

Measure	Finding	Points
	No gastrostomy; somewhat slow and clumsy but no help required	3
	No gastrostomy; can cut most foods although clumsy and slow; some help needed	2
	No gastrostomy; food must be cut by someone but can still feed slowly	1
	No gastrostomy; needs to be fed	0
	With gastrostomy; normal	4
	With gastrostomy; clumsy but able to perform all manipulations independently	3
	With gastrostomy; some help needed with closures and fasteners	2
	With gastrostomy; provides minimal assistance to caregiver	1
	With gastrostomy; unable to perform any aspect of task	0
Dressing and hygiene	Normal	4
	Independent and complete self-care with effort or decreased efficiency	3
	Intermittent assistance or substitute methods	2
	Needs attendant for self-care	1
	Total dependence	0
Turning in bed and adjusting bed clothes	Normal	4
	Somewhat slow and clumsy but no help needed	3
	Can turn alone or adjust sheets but with great difficulty	2
	Can initiate but not turn or adjust sheets alone	1
	Helpless	0
Walking	Normal	4
	Early ambulation difficulties	3
	Walks with assistance	2
	Nonambulatory functional movement only	1
	No purposeful leg movement	0
Climbing stairs	Normal	4
	Slow	3
	Mild unsteadiness or fatigue	2
	Needs assistance	1
	Cannot do	0

(continued)

Table 6.4 **Continued**

Measure	Finding	Points
Breathing	Normal	4
	Shortness of breath with minimal exertion (walking, talking, etc.)	3
	Shortness of breath at rest	2
	Intermittent (e.g., nocturnal) ventilatory assistance required	1
	Ventilator dependent	0

Source: Adapted from references 1 and 11.

At a later stage, healthcare workers in rehabilitation make use of the Functional Independence Measure (FIM score) that grades self-care, transfers, locomotion, and sphincter control,[19] (Chapter 2) but disability may already be defined by simple limitations such as inability to use arms (no buttoning, no tooth brushing or combing hair), inability to read clearly, frequent choking, and inability to walk stairs or arise from a chair. Fatigue after a long illness and a post intensive care (ICU) stress syndrome with irritability are all more or less hidden problems that may make life miserable for the patient and for the spouse pleased to finally see the much recovered patient returning home.

Long-term outcome measures have not been standardized in studies on acute neuromuscular disease but ability to wean from the ventilator is a crucial step (Figure 6.1).

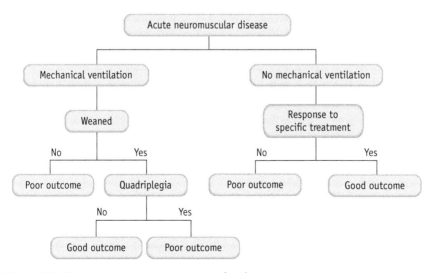

Figure 6.1 Outcome in acute neuromuscular disease.

In Practice

Four major disorders are typically cared for on the neurology ward or in the ICU. Over the years physicians have amassed sound empirical evidence of how these patients do over time. The outcome of these disorders is summarized here.

GUILLAIN-BARRÉ SYNDROME

Studies have shown that older age (>40 years), any preceding diarrhea, and severe weakness (low MRC sum score) on admission and one week after onset all predict a lower probability of walking not only within four weeks but also at three and six months.[33,44,53] Others have found that rapid disease progression (particularly within 3 days after onset of tingling), diarrhea with positive *Campylobacter jejuni* serology, positive cytomegalovirus serology, and the absence of a preceding common respiratory tract infection (indicating another antecedent event) predict poor outcome.[24,25,44,49] The acute motor axonal neuropathy variant of GBS is more prevalent in China, Japan, Bangladesh and South America. There is no associated pain or dysautonomia. Recovery may be rapid or slow and incomplete.[35]

Electrophysiology testing is able to determine the severity of nerve injury, whether motor responses are excitable, and whether fibrillations are widespread. These specific findings indicate severe demyelination with axonal involvement and are expected in a patient seen with rapid progression to quadriplegia and acute neuromuscular respiratory failure.[14] However, no electrophysiologic characteristic accurately predicts final outcome, and no hard predictions should be made on its appearance. Electrophysiology probably only provides a "snapshot in time." Certain electrophysiologic criteria such as a profound nerve conduction block or failure to obtain any nerve conduction velocity are only predictive of prolonged recovery, often months to years.

Prediction of respiratory failure is difficult at first presentation, but when there is a three-day interval between onset of weakness and hospital admission, presence of oropharyngeal weakness, and severe weakness in all extremities, respiratory failure is expected (a 90% chance).[54]

Once the patient is mechanically ventilated, a prolonged ICU stay is anticipated, with a high number of patients in need of a tracheostomy placement despite early administration of plasma exchange or IV immunoglobulin (IVIG). Still, about 75% of mechanically ventilated patients have regained the ability to walk independently, and the ability to become mobile may extend up to two years after onset.[13,17] Upper limb paralyses at peak disability may predict a lesser chance to ambulate. Nonetheless, patients may show clinically significant improvement beyond 1–2 years.[30] Intensive rehabilitation (most days of the week for 12 months) reduced disability in GBS and included less bladder and bowel problems along with improved motility and transfers.[30] It remains, however, impossible to predict who will stand up from a wheelchair and who will remain in a wheelchair, though again fortunately most will walk.[31,36,46] Mortality in GBS has been estimated at 3%, but doubles in long-term mechanically ventilated patients and may even approach 10%–20%.[17,36] Better ICU care and respiratory rehabilitation has greatly improved these percentages, but preexisting comorbidity (in particular prior lung disease) and the fragility of very old age remain disadvantages, and patients may succumb from an otherwise trivial pneumonitis.

MYASTHENIA GRAVIS

The age of onset is usually earlier in females than males, and myasthenia gravis presents in strange ways, always deceiving physicians. At onset patients may have several days of limb weakness followed by unnoticeable weakness for weeks, droopy eyes and transient ophthalmoparesis, and occasionally an oropharyngeal weakness or a dropping head. These presenting symptoms do not always indicate progression to generalization, although eventually many will get worse.

In ocular myasthenia, for example, about 50% of patients become generalized in 6 months, and that percentage increases to 80% in the next 2 years. If there are still only ocular symptoms 2 years from onset it will likely not worsen further. The outcome of myasthenia gravis is thus determined by whether the patient is affected by ocular symptoms or whether the disorder has led to more generalized symptoms. In most patients with myasthenia gravis, the disease severity becomes apparent within 6 months after onset. Most patients improve significantly after treatment. Approximately 10% of the patients will go into complete remission, less than 5% will worsen over time, and approximately 10% will die from the disorder or complications from the disorder.[6]

About 40% of the patients with generalized myasthenia gravis may develop a severe crisis at some point that requires endotracheal intubation and mechanical ventilation, mostly in the first two years from onset. The prognosis of myasthenia gravis may also be dependent on the presence of acute diaphragmatic failure and on timely therapy, with higher mortality in patients in whom plasma exchange was delayed for more than two days after presentation.

Thymectomy has had a significant effect on outcome, but it has never been a proven intervention.[2,3,20,38,39,48] Nonetheless, transsternal thymectomy is considered effective by many physicians who have seen the procedure increase the likelihood of remission.

Generally speaking, onset of myasthenia gravis in middle age has less severe manifestations, low probability of full remission, and higher mortality when compared with early-onset myasthenia. The worst outcome can be expected in patients with malignant thymoma, but only if the tumor has breached the capsule and caused metastasis.

The quality of life after myasthenia gravis is largely determined by the severity of muscle weakness (which may include weakness of neck muscles and constant head drop), dysphagia and chewing problems, ptosis, diplopia, and a speech impediment. Much of the quality of life is also influenced by the secondary effects of immunosuppressive therapy.[9] Outcome is thus dependent on choice of treatment and its long-term side effects.[18,23,39]

Overtime corticosteroids in high doses may cause the typical serious side effects such as hypertension, cataract, avascular hip necrosis, and osteoporosis.[40] Cyclosporine causes marked hypertension in susceptible patients and cannot always be adequately controlled. Other drugs such as mycophenolate mofetil, are associated with much less hypertension than cyclosporine, and have better tolerability.[55]

Depression is common in patients with myasthenia gravis.[34,47,50] It may be related to the significant expenditures on healthcare with multiple hospital admissions. Myasthenia gravis is a major chronic neurologic illness. Management by competent neurologists running specialized clinics should have better results for patients with long-standing myasthenia gravis.

AMYOTROPHIC LATERAL SCLEROSIS

Amyotrophic lateral sclerosis (ALS) will result in progressive shoulder and pectoral muscle wasting, atrophy in hand muscles (mostly first interossei and thenar muscles), and features of spasticity. Much of the wasting may be misinterpreted as weight loss, and some of it occurs when there is dysphagia and poor caloric intake. The emergence of widespread fasciculations will raise major concerns.

The outcome of ALS is approximately 3 years' survival in 50% of patients. One in 10 patients may live up to 10 years.[42,49] The patient with onset in limbs has a better outcome than patients with onset in the oropharyngeal region, and ALS starting in the legs has a slightly better outcome than that with early involvement of the arms.[21]

Survival after gastrostomy placement varies from 6 months to 42 months (median 12 months).[12] The onset of ALS with early respiratory involvement is not much different from that in patients with a bulbar onset and does not necessarily imply a much more progressive disease. Once respiration becomes involved in progressive ALS, the patient has a high likelihood of demise within a year unless mechanical ventilation is provided long-term. Conversely, many patients with ALS and normal pulmonary function tests do not require tracheostomy within 1 year.

The functional status of ventilated patients with ALS is quadriplegia in half of patients, some use of arms in a third, and communication with talking or mouthing of words and assisted communication (voice box) in many of them.

Management of respiratory symptoms is the most important determinant of outcome, and possible effective treatment includes reduction of excessive secretions (amitriptyline or scopolamine patches), avoidance of benzodiazepine and hypnotics, early gastrostomy tube placement to reduce aspiration, and the introduction of noninvasive ventilation.[41] A gastrostomy tube is often inserted if the patient is unable to maintain body weight or if there is frank dysphagia. When this procedure is performed patients may aspirate or have more difficulty breathing or handling secretions hours after the procedure. Additional use of noninvasive mechanical ventilation may reduce postoperative complications.[12]

Hypoxemia or hypercapnia is an important indication for noninvasive ventilation, and the vast majority are able to tolerate noninvasive ventilation quite well.[8,10,15,22,36,37] Noninvasive ventilation will improve both hypoxemia and hypercapnia, although it rarely normalizes these values. Some degree of hypoxemia and hypercapnia must be accepted.

Amyotrophic lateral sclerosis should be distinguished from primary lateral sclerosis (pyramidal signs only), progressive muscular atrophy (peripheral signs only), and progressive bulbar palsy (lower motor neuron involvement of speech and swallowing). Primary lateral sclerosis may have a median survival of 20 years, but the other disorders progress similarly to ALS. Outcome is also better in specialized clinics, largely due to much better symptom management.

CRITICAL ILLNESS POLYNEUROPATHY

Muscle mass is rapidly lost during critical illness, and due to proteolysis, nerve tissue can be damaged as well sometimes simultaneously. Both can lead to disability after surviving a critical illness.[43] Severe axonal polyneuropathy in patients who had sepsis or sepsis syndrome presents with symmetric, usually distal, limb weakness; areflexia and profound muscle weakness; and sometimes fasciculations. These patients usually have electrophysiologic findings of axonal polyneuropathy—many months are needed to improve. The outcome in critical illness neuropathy is entirely determined by the severity of sepsis and organ damage from septic syndrome. Septic encephalopathy might also play a role in rehabilitation, although this disorder is poorly defined and characterized. About one in five patients fail to significantly improve as a result of severe axonal destruction.

Critical illness polyneuropathy with myopathy is a very common neuromuscular disorder and has been increasingly recognized as a major health problem. Earlier observations were far more optimistic than more recent observations, and the disorder, particularly in an aging population, is very pertinent to resource utilization and physical activity. It is not known whether the complication increases mortality; but its presence prolongs time to discharge home, and long rehabilitation stays and effects may still be noticed 5 years from ICU discharge.[16,27]

By the Way

- Dysautonomia is rarely a cause of death in GBS
- Pure cholinergic causes are very uncommon in myasthenia gravis
- Respiratory symptoms in ALS may can be treated with noninvasive ventilation for many months
- Reintubation is common in myasthenia gravis, and many patients require a tracheostomy
- Poor functional status due to muscle or nerve tissue loss and weakness is common in survivors of sepsis

---

Acute Neuromuscular Disorders by the Numbers

- ~60% of patients with critical illness neuromyopathy may die from sepsis
- ~50% of patients with ALS die within 3 years
- ~40% of patients with myasthenia gravis develop a myasthenic crisis
- ~20% of patients with GBS are severely handicapped after 6 months
- ~10% of patients with myasthenia gravis die as a result of their disorder
- ~5% of patients with GBS die from medical complications

Putting It All Together

- Placement on a ventilator in acute neuromuscular disorders often defines outcome
- Functional independence may be difficult to gauge after an acute neuromuscular disease
- Many patients do well after GBS, but ambulation may take more than 6 months if upper extremities become paralyzed and mechanical ventilation is needed
- Short-term prognosis of myasthenia gravis is determined by a successful thymectomy and achievement of remission
- Long-term prognosis of myasthenia gravis is determined by complications of immunosuppressive therapy
- Care in ALS includes aggressive treatment of secretions, providing nutrition, and noninvasive ventilation

References

1. ALS CNTF Treatment Study (ACTS) Phase I-II Study Group. The Amyotrophic Lateral Sclerosis Functional Rating Scale. Assessment of activities of daily living in patients with amyotrophic lateral sclerosis. *Arch Neurol* 1996;53:141–147.

2. Bachmann K, Burkhardt D, Schreiter I, et al. Long-term outcome and quality of life after open and thoracoscopic thymectomy for myasthenia gravis: analysis of 131 patients. *Surg Endosc* 2008;22:2470–2477.

3. Bachmann K, Burkhardt D, Schreiter I, et al. Thymectomy is more effective than conservative treatment for myasthenia gravis regarding outcome and clinical improvement. *Surgery* 2009;145:392–398.

4. Barohn RJ, McIntire D, Herbelin L, et al. Reliability testing of the quantitative myasthenia gravis score. *Ann N Y Acad Sci* 1998;841:769–772.

5. Bedlack RS, Simel DL, Bosworth H, et al. Quantitative myasthenia gravis score: assessment of responsiveness and longitudinal validity. *Neurology* 2005;64:1968–1970.

6. Beghi E, Antozzi C, Batocchi AP, et al. Prognosis of myasthenia gravis: a multicenter follow-up study of 844 patients. *J Neurol Sci* 1991;106:213–220.

7. Bhanushali MJ, Wuu J, Benatar M. Treatment of ocular symptoms in myasthenia gravis. *Neurology* 2008;71:1335–1341.

8. Bourke SC, Bullock RE, Williams TL, Shaw PJ, Gibson GJ. Noninvasive ventilation in ALS: indications and effect on quality of life. *Neurology* 2003;61:171–177.

9. Burns TM. History of outcome measures for myasthenia gravis. *Muscle Nerve* 2010;42:5–13.

10. Caroscio JT, Calhoun WF, Yahr MD. Prognostic factors in motor neuron disease: a prospective study of longevity. In: Rose FC, ed. *Research Progress in Motor Neuron Disease*. London, Pitman, 1984, 34–43.

11. Cedarbaum JM, Stambler N. Performance of the Amyotrophic Lateral Sclerosis Functional Rating Scale (ALSFRS) in multicenter clinical trials. *J Neurol Sci* 1997;152:S1–S9.

12. Czell D, Bauer M, Binek J, et al. Outcome of percutaneous endoscopic gastrostomy tube insertion in respiratory impaired amyotrophic lateral sclerosis patients under non-invasive ventilation. *Respir Care* 2013;58:838–844.

13. Dhar R, Stitt L, Hahn AF. The morbidity and outcome of patients with Guillain-Barré syndrome admitted to the intensive care unit. *J Neurol Sci* 2008;264:121–128.

14. Durand MC, Lofaso F, Lefaucheur JP, et al. Electrophysiology to predict mechanical ventilation in Guillain-Barré syndrome. *Eur J Neurol* 2003;10:39–44.

15. Escarrabill J, Estopá R, Farrero E, Monasterio C, Manresa F. Long-term mechanical ventilation in amyotrophic lateral sclerosis. *Respir Med* 1998;92:438–441.

16. Fan E. Critical illness neuromyopathy and the role of physical therapy and rehabilitation in critically ill patients. *Respir Care* 2012;57:933–944; discussion 944–946.

17. Fletcher DD, Lawn ND, Wolter TD, Wijdicks EFM. Long-term outcome in patients with Guillain-Barré syndrome requiring mechanical ventilation. *Neurology* 2000;54:2311–2315.

18. Gajdos P, Chevret S. Treatment of myasthenia gravis acute exacerbations with intravenous immunoglobulin. *Ann N Y Acad Sci* 2008;1132:271–275.

19. Granger CV, Cotter AC, Hamilton BB, Fiedler RC, Hens MM. Functional assessment scales: a study of persons with multiple sclerosis. *Arch Phys Med Rehabil* 1990;71:870–875.

20. Grob D, Brunner N, Namba T, Pagala M. Lifetime course of myasthenia gravis. *Muscle Nerve* 2008;37:141–149.

21. Hardiman O, van den Berg LH, Kiernan MC. Clinical diagnosis and management of amyotrophic lateral sclerosis. *Nat Rev Neurol* 2011;7:639–649.

22. Haverkamp LJ, Appel V, Appel SH. Natural history of amyotrophic lateral sclerosis in a database population: validation of a scoring system and a model for survival prediction. *Brain* 1995;118:707–719.

23. Hehir MK, Burns TM, Alpers J, et al. Mycophenolate mofetil in AChR-antibody-positive myasthenia gravis: outcomes in 102 patients. *Muscle Nerve* 2010;41:593–598.

24. Henderson RD, Lawn ND, Fletcher DD, McClelland RL, Wijdicks EFM. The morbidity of Guillain-Barré syndrome admitted to the intensive care unit. *Neurology* 2003;60:17–21.

25. Hughes RAC, Cornblath DR. Guillain-Barré syndrome. *Lancet* 2005;366:1653–1666.

26. Hughes RAC, Wijdicks EFM, Benson E, et al. Supportive care for patients with Guillain-Barré syndrome. *Arch Neurol* 2005;62:1194–1198.

27. Intiso D, Amoruso L, Zarrelli M, et al. Long-term functional outcome and health status of patients with critical illness polyneuromyopathy. *Acta Neurol Scand* 2011;123:211–219.

28. Jaretzki A 3rd, Barohn RJ, Ernstoff RM, et al; Task Force of the Medical Scientific Advisory Board of the Myasthenia Gravis Foundation of America. Myasthenia gravis: recommendations for clinical research standards. *Neurology* 2000;55:16–23.

29. Khan F, Ng L, Amatya B, Brand C, Turner-Stokes L. Multidisciplinary care for Guillain-Barré syndrome. *Cochrane Database Syst Rev* 2010;CD008505.

30. Khan F, Pallant JF. Use of the International Classification of Functioning, Disability and Health to identify preliminary comprehensive and brief core sets for Guillain Barre syndrome. *Disabil Rehabil* 2011;33:1306–1313.

31. Khan F, Pallant JF, Amatya B, et al. Outcomes of high- and low-intensity rehabilitation programme for persons in chronic phase after Guillain-Barré syndrome: a randomized controlled trial. *J Rehabil Med* 2011;43:638–646.

32. Khan F, Pallant JF, Ng L, Bhasker A. Factors associated with long-term functional outcomes and psychological sequelae in Guillain-Barre syndrome. *J Neurol* 2010;257:2024–2031.

33. Köhrmann M, Huttner HB, Nowe T, Schellinger PD, Schwab S. Mechanical ventilation in Guillain-Barré syndrome: does age influence functional outcome? *Eur Neurol* 2009;61:358–363.

34. Kulaksizoglu IB. Mood and anxiety disorders in patients with myasthenia gravis: etiology, diagnosis and treatment. *CNS Drugs* 2007;21:473–481.

35. Kuwabara S, Yuki N. Axonal Guillain-Barré syndrome: concepts and controversies. *Lancet Neurol* 2013;12:1180–1188.

36. Lawn ND, Wijdicks EFM. Fatal Guillain-Barré syndrome. *Neurology* 1999;52:635–638.

37. Louwerse ES, Visser CE, Bossuyt PMM, Weverling GJ, and the Netherlands ALS Consortium. Amyotrophic lateral sclerosis: mortality risk during the course of the disease and prognostic factors. *J Neurol Sci* 1997;152:S10–S17.

38. Maggi L, Andreetta F, Antozzi C, et al. Thymoma-associated myasthenia gravis: outcome, clinical and pathological correlations in 197 patients on a 20-year experience. *J Neuroimmunol* 2008;201–202:237–244.

39. Mandawat A, Mandawat A, Kaminski HJ, Shaker ZA, et al. Outcome of plasmapheresis in myasthenia gravis: delayed therapy is not favorable. *Muscle Nerve* 2011;43:578–584.

40. Mann JD, Johns TR, Campa JF. Long-term administration of corticosteroids in myasthenia gravis. *Neurology* 1976;26:729–740.

41. Miller RG, Jackson CE, Kasarskis EJ, et al. Practice parameter update: the care of the patient with amyotrophic lateral sclerosis: drug, nutritional, and respiratory therapies (an evidence-based review): report of the Quality Standards Subcommittee of the American Academy of Neurology. *Neurology* 2009;73:1218–1226.

42. Norris F, Sheperd R, Denys E, et al. Onset, natural history and outcome in idiopathic adult motor neuron disease. *J Neurol Sci* 1993;118:48–55.

43. Puthucheary ZA, Rawal J, McPhail M, et al. Acute skeletal muscle wasting in critical illness. *JAMA* 2013;310:1591–1600.

44. Rajabally YA, Uncini A. Outcome and its predictors in Guillain-Barre syndrome. *J Neurol Neurosurg Psychiatry* 2012;83:711–718.

45. Ropper AH, Kehne SM. Guillain-Barré syndrome: management of respiratory failure. *Neurology* 1985;35:1662–1665.

46. Ropper AH. Severe acute Guillain-Barré syndrome. *Neurology* 1986;36:429–432.

47. Scott KR, Kothari MJ. Self-reported pain affects quality of life in myasthenia gravis. *J Clin Neuromuscul Dis* 2006;7:110–114.

48. Takanami I, Abiko T, Koizumi S. Therapeutic outcomes in thymectomied patients with myasthenia gravis. *Ann Thorac Cardiovasc Surg* 2009;15:373–377.

49. Testa D, Lovati R, Ferrarini M, Salmoiraghi F, Filippini G. Survival of 793 patients with amyotrophic lateral sclerosis diagnosed over a 28-year period. *Amyotrophic Lateral Sclerosis* 2004;5:208–212.

50. Twork S, Wiesmeth S, Klewer J, Pöhlau D, Kugler J. Quality of life and life circumstances in German myasthenia gravis patients. *Health Qual Life Outcomes* 2010;8:129.
51. Van Doorn PA, Ruts L, Jacobs BC. Clinical features, pathogenesis, and treatment of Guillain-Barré syndrome. *Lancet Neurol* 2008;7:939–950.
52. Vanhoutte EK, Faber CG, van Nes SI, et al. Modifying the Medical Research Council grading system through Rasch analyses. *Brain* 2012;135:1639–1649.
53. Walgaard C, Lingsma HF, Ruts L, et al. Early recognition of poor prognosis in Guillain-Barre syndrome. *Neurology* 2011;76:968–975.
54. Walgaard C, Lingsma HF, Ruts L, et al. Prediction of respiratory insufficiency in Guillain-Barré syndrome. *Ann Neurol* 2010;67:781–787.
55. Wolfe GI, Barohn RJ, Sanders DB, McDermott MP; Muscle Study Group. Comparison of outcome measures from a trial of mycophenolate mofetil in myasthenia gravis. *Muscle Nerve* 2008;38:1429–1433.

7

Principles of Neuropalliation

The distress of being in an intensive care unit is substantial, with discomfort from nasogastric and endotracheal tubes, repeated blood draws, and symptoms of pain, fear, and agitation. Moreover, very few acutely ill neurologic patients are able to communicate the level of care desired. The acute stress facing family members is enormous. However, objectionable as it may sound, acute neurology cannot be understood as a specialty of curing illnesses. We all know that patients may do very well after aggressive intervention, and for physicians and nursing staff there are many moments of relief, but acute severe neurologic illness with poor outcome is common. In these patients, decisions on the degree of care are very often made in intensive care settings, where for many families advanced technology now may seem "normal" and there for the right reasons—to improve outcome. De-escalation or palliation may incorrectly come across as "giving up."

Who has the power to decide and what determines the level of care? Most of us dread a poor neurologic outcome, particularly if the outcome is nothing other than sustaining life. There are contrasting positions. On one side (definitely extreme) is the vitalist argument emphasizing life and its sanctity and a philosophy that deemphasizes the patient's autonomy. The other position holds a utilitarian (or perhaps secular humanist) view emphasizing privacy and autonomy. Many positions are somewhere in between and a continuum may exist.

Despite these philosophical questions, there has been a recent major cultural shift in clinical practice: a change in the approach to family members, with the main focus on what the patient wants.[18,21] In the United States and many other countries, physicians practice a family-centered approach to palliation. The ultimate goal is to provide what is euphemistically called a "good death." The true goal of this approach is to ensure that the patient is not abandoned, not suffering, comfortable, and with a resigned understanding—and not acrimonious—family.[2,4]

To provide solace and adequate neuropalliation is a major task. Neurologists (neurohospitalists and neurointensivists) have the opportunity to build up an extensive experience in these interactions, to respect human dignity, to appreciate autonomy and individual rights, and to become trained in end-of-life communication.[5]

Therefore, the final chapters of this book are entirely focused on the practical support of the dying neurologic patient and family. Questions to address here are: Is neuropalliation different from palliation in patients with an incurable medical illness? Can palliation in neurologic patients who cannot communicate be based on more than inference? What are the core principles of neuroethics? This chapter introduces some of the commonly encountered ethical quandaries.

Principles

The principles of neuropalliation include major bioethical decisions. The World Health Organization has defined palliative care as "an approach that improves the quality of life of patients and their families facing the problem associated with life-threatening illness," and it specifically emphasizes several attributes: "palliative care provides relief of pain and other distressing symptoms; affirms life and regards dying as a normal process; intends neither to hasten nor postpone death; integrates the psychological and spiritual aspects of care; offers a support system for family and patient; offers bereavement counseling; and understands that it can be applicable early in the course of the illness in conjunction with other therapies intended to prolong life." The American Academy of Neurology, the American Medical Association, and other major medical organizations in Europe and the U.K. have made similar statements.

Palliative care is not solely seen as comfort care in the terminal phase only. Palliative care may involve surgical procedures to relieve pain or to provide access to nutrition. Palliative care could involve radiotherapy and neurosurgical procedures. Removal of a metastasis causing obstructive hydrocephalus, or more specific procedures to relieve pain are some examples. Futile neurosurgical procedures may be hard to define, and empirical judgment in each situation is needed. Neurosurgeons would consider an operation only if it would reduce suffering and likely will have the potential to improve quality of care.

PRIMER OF NEUROETHICS

The core principles of neuroethics are closely related to the basics of bioethics. The first core principle is to apply the fundamentals of medical ethics, dominated by the four principles of Beauchamp and Childress outlined in their textbook *Principles of Biomedical Ethics*. These are autonomy, nonmaleficence, beneficence, and justice. These principles have been important pillars in many problematic and difficult cases and, according to the authors, have equal importance. Every physician is now asked to interpret these definitions and voice them to the family members and the patient in their own language in understandable and unambiguous terms (Table 7.1).

The first pillar is autonomy. Generally speaking, autonomy overrides beneficence. This means that even if there is a potential for benefit, the patient may

Table 7.1 **Common Bioethical Terms**

Term	Explanation
Autonomy	Patient or family decides
Beneficence	Do what is best
Nonmaleficence	Do no harm and avoid harm
Justice	Fairness and all treated the same
Conflict of interest	Withdrawal of support may have other intent
Coercion	Imposing will on patient
Paternalism	Doctor knows best

refuse all medical intervention. In principle, autonomy refers to a patient's ability to make a choice; however, it also applies to a physician making a choice. Physicians cannot be forced to make a certain decision, nor do patients have to be forced to proceed along a certain pathway. Autonomy is closely linked to competence and the ability to make a choice, understand the condition, and grapple with the reasons for medical treatment. The major challenge for neurologists is to remain unbiased respect the patient's decisions and not consider them irrational. Patients have the right to be informed, the right to refuse or consent, and the right to have directives written in advance. Patients can also waive the right to know.

In a patient with acute neurologic illness information can be extracted from advance directives where the patient's wishes are stated, or decisions are relegated to spouse or next of kin. How often physicians respect the autonomy of the patient remains unknown and could be unsettling in some practices. Autonomy of the patient is markedly challenged if physicians use manipulation or coercion, which may include pushing for do-not-resuscitate (DNR) orders or withdrawal of support. The physician does not have the privilege to change a DNR order without the patient's or family's consent and should always document the reasons for doing so. At the other extreme is the decision to simply ignore repeated requests for de-escalating care. For example, to proceed with withdrawal of care only when the one-month threshold has been passed raises concerns (most US institutions use one month as the benchmark for postoperative mortality).

The second pillar, beneficence, is defined as balancing the benefits against the risks. Many physicians see the concept of beneficence as the principle of improving quality of life, and consider prolonging life to be justified only if it has the potential to improve quality of life. The third pillar is nonmaleficence, which simply indicates avoiding harm. Harm may be seen from a patient perspective (unnecessary continuation of treatment) or from a physician perspective (providing treatment that could clearly worsen the patient). Of course no physician should even think of causing harm to the patient, but the fact is that harm to the patient and family may be far more subtle. One could argue that harm may even mean mounting large medical bills (which have the potential to bankrupt a patient's family) in pursuit of an aggressive treatment in a futile situation. Harm may also include causing major side effects from useless interventions that may appear acceptable to the family but only because there is the perception that the physician is doing all he can.

The fourth pillar is justice, and implies avoidance of unfair and discriminatory decisions. Justice is a principle that is more easily debated than carried out at the bedside. In the hospital there should be timeliness of care and full access irrespective of age, insurance status, comorbidity, or lifestyle. Therefore, with this principle, a chronic alcoholic or reckless patient with major self-inflicted comorbidities or recent injury should receive healthcare similar to that received by a patient with a chosen life of wellness. Any vulnerable member of the community should be protected in accord with the principle of fair equality of opportunity. There should be no discrimination and avoidance of discriminatory language toward an ethnically different population. Justice ensures that the patient receives the best opportunity for treatment available. Of course, variations in healthcare between hospitals, and variations of skill on the part of physicians and other healthcare workers, make this technically an illusion.

A fifth pillar of neuroethics must be confidentiality. Physicians should have the patient or family decide who can be informed and who cannot. In acute neurologic conditions most patients are unaware of their illness. In this situation, disclosure of personal information to family members is necessary despite the lack of patient consent. In this situation, family members should be able to trust the physician to keep all information private and within the circle of those involved with patient care.

A second core principle is to maximize quality of life and dignity.[7,8,9,17,20,22] There is no satisfactory definition of "dignity." The term probably incorporates normalcy, respect, and personal appearance. To honor dignity, physicians should ensure that comfort, adequate pain control, and uninterrupted care are provided.[10,14,16,17,19]

Families often summarize lack of dignity best when they state, "He doesn't want to live like this." Their loved one is now on a mechanical ventilator and fed through a gastrostomy tube, facial features have changed dramatically, and he or she has become unrecognizable to family members. Being continuously supported by machines after a neurologic catastrophe does increase the likelihood of a patient's quality of life being characterized as demoralizing and hopeless. "Independence" is a far more nebulous and uninterpretable term, but its absence undermines a sense of personal pride. However, some caregivers may be convinced that they can ensure that the patient does not feel burdensome, ensure well being and they may feel it is "just the right thing to do" to continue all possible care.

A third core principle is to appreciate an increasingly global world. Patients and families may come from different cultural or religious backgrounds. This may introduce unorthodox perceptions of illness and even differences of opinion with the physician about whether details of illness should be disclosed to the patient or proxy in the first place. Emotional expressions vary in different cultures and may be appropriate to one and very inappropriate to others. Race and ethnicity may be also drive certain types of decisions.[15] Families who are less aware of the limitations of medicine may be more eager to "try everything." This demands respect in many situations. There are also different bereavement practices according to differing cultural backgrounds.

Physicians should ward against stereotyping and inform themselves about the nature of the patient's beliefs. Because each faith tradition has its own rituals, religious worship in the hospital should be provided if requested. Religion has a major effect on healthcare, and patients and families are more likely to be religious than not. For both families and patients, faith may provide a coping strategy, hope in after-life, and belief in divine intervention that allows healing (not necessarily a cure). But religious beliefs at times may harm (not allowing essential interventions), obstruct (not allowing withdrawal of care), or cause resentment and helplessness (when prayers are not answered.)

In the United States, there is a major heterogeneity in religion. In Europe, Anglo-Saxon, North European, and Mediterranean traditions predominate, but laws usually determine decisions. In many Asian countries, treatment withdrawal is not generally accepted as a compassionate practice, and many family members will often profess their belief that continuation of care is always acceptable and needed.

Generally speaking, neuropalliation for devastating neurologic disorders has been accepted by all major religions. But patient's families may have different ideas colored by cultural attitudes, traditional customs, and personal beliefs.[22] The major religions in the United States include Christianity, Islam, and Judaism, and often they are divided into various denominations. Islam is the religion of Muslims, and the traditional teaching is that Muslims should not give up, which implies that termination of life support is not allowed. The prophet Muhammad said that God has not created a disease without a cure, and Muslims believe that all diseases can be cured if it is God's will. For Muslims, death is a path to another, everlasting life. Islamic medical jurisprudence is, however, in favor of declaring brain death as the death of a person.

The Jewish law (Halacha) is dependent on rabbinic opinions. Generally, the Jewish tradition emphasizes that alleviation of suffering is a duty. There is a general belief that death can be a blessing for the patient and that it is a path to eternal existence. The definition of death is controversial. More conservative branches have, over the years, rejected any classification of death other than by respiratory and circulatory criteria. The orthodox Jewish community in New York has been successful in lobbying for a religious exception to the New York statute regarding brain death. In New York and New Jersey, a devout Orthodox Jew can demand that the attending physician continue support and respect their religious belief that cardiac arrest is the only sign of death. However, relatively few rabbis still follow the ancient teachings that define cardiac arrest as the defining moment of death.

The beliefs of Christian denominations are rooted in the Bible. Actively hastening death for some violates the commandments of God. Christians have faith in miracles, but do not expect a miracle if physicians communicate a hopeless situation. Many Christian denominations see withdrawal of care and removal of a nasogastric tube in a futile situation as acceptable, though some see it as active killing. Clergy can play an important role in explaining the clinical situation and church dogma.

Christian denominations interpret brain death as the death of a person and feel that organ donation is the ultimate gift of life. There is no controversy in the Catholic Church or with any other denominations. The Roman Catholic Church legitimizes organ donation by the principle of solidarity and charity. It is permissible to remove the life support system if attending specialist physicians render their opinion unequivocally that irreversible cessation of brain functions has occurred.

There might be a personal conviction of the family that the patient is not dead, which may lead to a conflict between the family and the physician. When this occurs, legal counsel is advised, but, at least in the United States, there is no legal obligation to continue care of a person that has been declared dead.

Both the Chinese and Japanese have cultural value systems that do not, as in Western cultures, emphasize self-determination. Many spiritual movements, including Taoism, prevalent in China, have not expressed opinions on long-term care, and a considerable amount of diversity is expected.

In many religions there is surely some discomfort with performing an autopsy or removing organs. In some cultures it is difficult to obtain consent from families for organ donation. Some families question whether an incomplete body may go to heaven or be resurrected. In an attempt to resolve this matter, physicians have emphasized that many persons die by fire or destructive accidents, and cremations are commonly performed.

In Practice

The first important assessment is whether the patient has decision-making capacity. The important elements of capacity for decision-making are the ability to communicate a choice, the capability of making a reasonable treatment choice, the understanding of the importance and the meaning of the decision, and appreciation of the consequences. Any adult should have the most appropriate information available, and it should be communicated understandably.

This may be very difficult with a patient and an acute brain injury who is confused, agitated, or unresponsive and uncommunicative. Generally, when providing information physicians also need to clearly address alternative options. An adult patient who is informed and has adequate decision-making capacity should be allowed to forego any life-sustaining therapy, even if it would result in rapid respiratory and cardiac arrest. In US courts, it is accepted that artificial nutrition and hydration, whether provided by oral, nasal or percutaneous feeding tube, is a medical intervention. Therefore, there are no legal distinctions between withholding and withdrawing. When the patient is unable to make decisions, a surrogate decision-maker must decide for the patient. When a surrogate decision-maker cannot be reached and there is an emergency, physicians will have to make the decisions for the patient. Surrogate decisionmakers may be legally established with a durable power of attorney, and, in some instances, this may not necessarily be a member of the patient's family. Any surrogate decision-maker could make a decision based on the patient's best interest and judge benefits of treatment versus burdens of treatment. A family that decides to continue aggressive care in a severely brain-injured patient with significant comorbidity should understand the probability of a long road of infections, the possibility of skin breakdown, need for pain control, total dependency, and the certainty of no quality of life.

Physicians are obliged to relieve pain. Since the common problem of a drug's effect on a patient diminishes over time, return of pain may not imply progression of the disease. Tolerance does develop to the side effects of opioids, including respiratory depression and nausea. Judging pain in a patient with an abnormal level of consciousness is difficult, but groaning, agitation, diaphoresis, hypertension, and unexplained tachycardia with movement of the patient might indicate pain that justifies pain medication. Palliative interventional pain therapy is important in noncomatose patients. There is no evidence, to support the use of sedatives or analgesics in patients who are comatose, and such use may be misunderstood as uncertainty on the part of the physician about whether there is pain perception. Using sedatives or analgesics "just to be sure" is poor practice. A commonly used term here is "proportionality." This indicates that the physician's response to a certain degree of suffering is justified and does not create a higher risk of hastening the patient's death. If patients are not responding to a significant dose of narcotics, a higher dose can be used to better treat the patient without insinuating a bad intention.[1] A commonly used example of poor practice is continuing narcotics in high dose and not adjusting the medication after relief of the targeted symptoms.

Treatment limitations are very frequent in hospitals in the developed world. At that time, it has been determined that the patient is at the end of life. These above mentioned interventions are legally justified, even though aggressive palliation could potentially hasten the patient's death—a very uncommon occurrence. This is not considered assisted suicide or euthanasia, because the intent (pain control) is utterly different. Generally, the patient's family and physician decide how much suffering is too much for a dying patient.[2]

There are three ways to provide end-of-life care, although their definitions have been much debated. A reasonable definition is necessary to come to a general understanding of what these decisions entail.

The first is assisted suicide, which is a clinician facilitating the death of the patient by providing the means. This may also consist of providing information on how to obtain the means, and this may also include instructions. Usually it involves a prescription of medication. The patient performs the act that results in death. There is clear understanding that the prescription is for the patient's intent to die. Assisted suicide is illegal in the United States, except in Oregon. It is legal in the Benelux countries in Europe and illegal in all Asian countries.

The second is euthanasia, the administration by a physician of a drug that immediately causes death. This is illegal in every state in the United States, but is legal in several European countries. In these countries, there is no distinction between these two forms of assisted dying, whether it is by the patient (assisted suicide) or by the physician (euthanasia). The procedure typically involves administration of a neuromuscular blocker and sedative agent in combination. There have been published guidelines and strict protocols in countries where this procedure is allowed.

The third is withholding or withdrawing interventions or withholding support. Physicians should not be forced to proceed with withdrawal of care if they feel it is not appropriate in that particular situation. What can be said is that when a proxy decision-maker is unclear about the patient's preferences, it is best to err on the side of continuing care. This is perhaps the most difficult situation; the physician often cannot guarantee a successful outcome, and often a certain period of time is needed to come to a conclusion that further treatment is inappropriate.[11]

With this intervention, the patient is not provided a high level of medical care; as a result of that, the patient may die. It is clearly considered a de-escalation of care in a patient with an irreversible, hopeless condition, whereas aggressive support is seen as an interruption or prolonging of the dying process. Withdrawal of care often also requires active comfort care.[6] For example in end-stage ALS, physicians should treat dyspnea but also should explain that this is not a sign of choking to death and symptoms can be treated appropriately.[3] These patients do not die from lack of air intake, and suffocation is not a consequence of progressive neurologic disease. Withholding may also be initiated by the family. This approach is overwhelmingly accepted by physicians and the public. Essential in making these decisions is that patients or proxy have a decisional capacity and that there is no indication of coercion. Withdrawal of food and hydration from comatose patients is usually not considered controversial, although there has been objection against these practices. Despite these objections, the case of Terri Schiavo and other cases of persistent vegetative state have led to no major change in US legislation. In other countries, hydration and feeding might be considered mandatory and, in some countries (e.g., Germany and Austria), there is a subtle distinction between limiting treatments, implying no treatment of infections or complications, and withdrawal of treatment, implying withdrawal of mechanical ventilation.

When do we consider transition to palliative care? Advance directives may have outlined a refusal of further treatment in a specific situation, but they may not correspond with the patient's best interest. For example, a patient with a treatable lobar hematoma and a DNR order would benefit from a neurosurgical procedure and might die if not treated. If the patient's family continues to refuse, the circumstances in which the refusal applies should be documented.

There is a professional duty of physicians to aid families and patients when end-of-life decisions have been made. This process involves a gradual institution of palliative care, or a sudden transition (Figure 7.1). A gradual model allows hospital palliative services to weigh in. Unfortunately, the experience of palliative care services is that more than 70% of patients are moribund, suggesting earlier involvement could have been instigated.

Physicians known that patients are vulnerable in their relationship and reliant on the physician for treatment. Communication with family must be

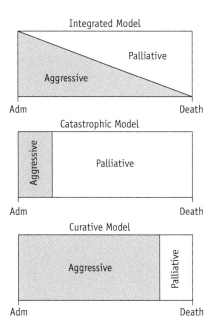

Figure 7.1 Models of care and different ways of integrating aggressive care with palliative care.

established at a sufficient level that what needs to be said is not only said to them but also accepted and understood by them.

This part of acute neurology is difficult, and not everyone takes to it naturally. To be constantly and assertively clarifying the reality to patients and patients' families easily takes a toll. Being frequently involved with neuropalliation leads to burn-out and a phenomenon called compassion fatigue (a possible variant of post-traumatic stress syndrome) that brings with it avoidance behavior, reexperiencing patients' suffering, emotional exhaustion, a sense of ineffectiveness, and social withdrawal.[13] With each day bringing bad news, discouragement, long discussions on the futility of care, and supporting families, physicians need personal coping skills, good insights and often a break from it all.

If the family fails to accept the futility of care, the physician should consider maintaining full support and, in turn, asking for assistance from a hospital ethics committee and perhaps spiritual counsel. Physicians should appreciate these sensitivities and try to help family members reach a sense of closure. Continuing support should be full support, and it is poor practice to maintain mechanical ventilation and just a minimal level of other interventions, effectively hastening cardiac arrest.

If the family refuses to come to an agreement and remains intransigent, legal advice can be obtained. On rare occasions, families may request that certain rituals be performed. Such a request could generally be honored unless it is an attempt to change the medical condition. One request may also be followed by other requests, which could lead to prolonged continued care in a patient who has no chance of improvement.

By the Way

- Medication and pain may impact patient's decisions.
- Futility is difficult to assess
- Communication with intubated patient may be unreliable
- Patients with poor prognosis should not have care escalated
- When full code is requested, full code should be provided

Neuropalliation by the Numbers

- ~90% of patients feel that being a burden determines level of care
- ~70% of families in the US request spiritual support
- ~70% of decisions in NICU to limit care occur within 3 days
- ~20% of neurologic patients in the United States die in the ICU
- ~20% of neurologic patients in NICU are capable of making a decision

Putting It All Together

- Palliative care should be integrated in the education of neurohospitalists
- Palliative care strives to provide good quality of life near the end of life
- Attempts to prolong life and palliative treatment can occur at the same time
- Cultural attitudes can be barriers to optimal palliative care
- Physicians should avoid interventions that prolong suffering

References

1. Alvarez A, Walsh D. Symptom control in advanced cancer: twenty principles. *Am J Hosp Palliat Care* 2011;28:203–207.
2. Angell, M. The right to death. *New York Review of Books.* 2012 Nov 8.
3. Arras JD. Getting down to cases: the revival of casuistry in bioethics. *J Med Philos* 1991;16:29–51.
4. Balducci L. Death and dying: what the patient wants. *Ann Oncol* 2012;23:56–61.
5. Bede P, Oliver D, Stodart J, et al. Palliative care in amyotrophic lateral sclerosis: a review of current international guidelines and initiatives. *J Neurol Neurosurg Psychiatry* 2011;82:413–418.
6. Brennan CW, Prince-Paul M, Wiencek CA. Providing a "good death" for oncology patients during the final hours of life in the intensive care unit. *AACN Adv Crit Care* 2011;22:379–396.
7. Campbell ML, Weissman DE, Nelson JE. Palliative care consultation in the ICU #253. *J Palliat Med* 2012;15:715–716.
8. Chochinov HM, Hack T, Hassard T, Kristjanson LJ, McClement S, Harlos M. Dignity in the terminally ill: a cross-sectional, cohort study. *Lancet* 2002;360:2026–2030.
9. Chochinov HM, Krisjanson LJ, Hack TF, Hassard T, McClement S, Harlos M. Dignity in the terminally ill: revisited. *J Palliat Med* 2006;9:666–672.
10. Dickie B. Defining the principles of palliative care in amyotrophic lateral sclerosis. *J Neurol Neurosurg Psychiatry* 2011;82:356.
11. Faber-Langendoen K, Bartels DM. Process of forgoing life-sustaining treatment in a university hospital: an empirical study. *Crit Care Med* 1992;20:570–577.
12. Foster C. Putting dignity to work. *Lancet* 2012;379:2044–2045.
13. Kearney MK, Weininger RB, Vachon MLS, et al. Self-care of physicians caring for patients at the end of life. *JAMA* 2009;30:1155–1164.
14. Macklin R. Dignity is a useless concept. *BMJ* 2003;327:1419–1420.

15. McKinley ED, Garrett JM, Evans AT, Danis M. Differences in end-of-life decision making among black and white ambulatory cancer patients. *J Gen Intern Med* 1996;11:651–656.

16. McMenamin E. Pain management principles. *Curr Probl Cancer* 2011;35:317–324.

17. O'Dowd A. Review calls for major changes to care of older people to restore dignity. *BMJ* 2012;344:e4214.

18. Ostlund U, Brown H, Johnston B. Dignity conserving care at end-of-life: a narrative review. *Eur J Oncol Nurs* 2012;16:353–367.

19. Page K. The four principles: Can they be measured and do they predict ethical decision making? *BMC Med Ethics* 2012;13:10.

20. Quill TE. Death and dignity. A case of individualized decision making. *N Engl J Med* 1991; 324:691–694.

21. Seymour J. Changing times: preparing to meet palliative needs in the 21st Century. *Br J Community Nurs* 2011;16:18.

22. Sulmasy DP. Ethos, mythos, and tanathos: spirituality and ethics at the end of life. *J Pain Symptom Manage* 2013;46:447–451.

8

The Conversation and Words We Use

Patients who are stricken by an acute severe neurologic injury may follow several clinical trajectories; some of these pathways may be clear and others are less certain. These patients and those near to them are suddenly confronted with a new situation and the realization that their lives have suddenly changed forever. Any neurologist might at any time have to honestly and openly discuss the consequences of acute neurologic disease.

As emphasized in Chapter 7, to discuss the patient's condition with family members requires a focus on one major goal: to honor the patient's assumed wishes.[7,8,9] However, the way neurologists describe the current neurologic condition has an immediate impact on decision-making, because many families will follow the neurologist's lead. Moderating such a family conference therefore requires skill, patience, and perhaps even decades of experience.[52,56]

This family conference should be structured in such a way that it will be realistic and productive. How do we best understand the families' sensitivities? How can we lead a cordial exchange of medical facts and expectations? How can family conferences go amiss? How do we recognize misgivings about the outcome? This chapter covers bedside manners, methodology of discussion, and, above all, how to provide a measured response to end-of-life questions.

Principles

A major component in discussions with the families of such patients is the neurologist's personal traits and qualities. Empathy or compassion are necessary. Compassion is defined by the *Oxford English Dictionary* as "sympathetic pity and concern for the sufferings or misfortunes of others." The word is derived from the Latin *compassio*, from *compati*, or "suffer with." Compassion may be a personality trait and perhaps cannot be taught. Maybe maturity and frequent patient interactions can teach compassion, but some physicians never lose a paternalistic inclination and look nonplussed when criticized. No physician can tell another physician how to be compassionate or how to empathetically care for patients. Nonetheless, one could look critically at behavior and change behavior, deconstruct compassion, look at errors made, and perhaps even explain empathy during early training.[52]

The four major elements of compassion are accountability, honesty, authenticity, and genuineness.[41,42,48,53,57] Accountability pertains to bringing sufficient knowledge to a constructive discussion with family members. To express excessive confidence in one's own judgments, however, is a mistake. Patients and families need to know—and expect—that we are imperfect.[30] Moreover, wavering and peppering the conversation with medical terms is better replaced by explaining what is known and what is absolutely not known.

Another way of looking at compassion is to look at what might not be compassionate. There are some common behavioral elements displayed by physicians who lack compassion.[10,34] These may start with presenting themselves unshaven after call, inappropriately answering pages, failing to give families undivided attention, or refraining from eye contact. In the introduction to family members, failure to explain the role and specialty and failure to identify family members or how they are related, will immediately diminish the trustworthiness of the physician. Some physicians have a tendency to speak in third person or use the "royal we," and this may be confusing to family members. Posture is also important. Standing, leaning against the wall, or sitting restlessly in a swivel chair are not only unprofessional but also may be interpreted as lack of compassion. Arrogance can be recognized by certain mimicry, impulsiveness, using terms such as "in my experience," and monotonic, businesslike modulation of speech. The phrase "I am so very sorry" is important, but must be used at the appropriate moment.[5,26] When communication is performed in a scripted, mechanical, and depersonalized manner, conflicts arise; the principle of joint decision-making may disappear quickly, and family/neurologist discord (Chapter 10) may emerge and even lead to litigation.

Adequate compassion includes coaching, assistance, and support for families while they are preparing for a period of bereavement. Maintaining hope is also part of compassion.[19,28] Neurologists should allow long periods of silence if that is the most appropriate way of handling a difficult situation. Compassion also involves being candid, as concealment of information will always lead to immediate distrust. Exaggerations should be avoided. Phrases such as "I am fighting for the patient," "we're doing all we can," or "we just pulled him back off the brink" are not only inaccurate but also quite inappropriate and aggrandizing. Most family members easily recognize hubristic behavior.[34]

One of the first core principles is to provide factual information. A guide for a comprehensive conversation is shown in Table 8.1. This is best done in a separate place that allows all involved to sit down. Many physicians still may have these discussions right outside of the patient's room, but unless this is done to discuss simple issues or to clarify a simple concern, standing outside a room is not an ideal situation for discussing large matters and is not sufficiently private. The key persons who should be present are family, next of kin, the decision-maker and power of attorney (if available in the family), clergy (if warranted), representatives of the nursing staff, and social workers. Communication with the family takes time and requires an attempt to explore the family's understanding of the patient's preferences. One person

Table 8.1 **A Structure for Conversations with the Patient's Family**

- Gather all close members and the person with power of attorney (if relevant)
- Spend at least 30 minutes
- Have nursing staff, clergy, social work, and other consultants present
- Discuss "the big picture"
- Discuss what the patient is noticing
- Discuss what the patient would want under these circumstances
- Discuss current plan
- Discuss medical and neurosurgical options
- Discuss best estimate of outcome
- Discuss timeline of improvement, if any
- Discuss code status and resuscitation efforts
- Set up follow-up meeting

should be identified as the person who leads the conversation. Understandably, this is the neurologist, but the nursing staff caring for the patient should provide valuable information in explaining the condition of the patient.

After an update of the clinical course, the neurologist should almost immediately explain the big picture. This includes not only the current treatment plan but also a more careful explanation of options. Neurologists may need to use CT scans to point to the injury and to discuss what it means.

Decisions should never be made by neurologists alone or families alone. Early on, it is important to explain directly to all involved that one of the other important goals of the conference is to achieve a mutual agreement also-called "shared decision-making."[4,55] This nebulous term implies making decisions that are shared between neurologists and families, and decisions made with input from both. Such a process also implies a remarkable four-way understanding between patient, family, nursing staff, and physician. This may be straightforward if the family agrees with the physician and the prior wishes of the patient are perfectly known. This model does not put the onus on the family but simply informs them. The decision is a reflection of patient's wishes—in other words—what could the patient have decided if he or she would be able to tell. However—and here it becomes dicey—there is is not much to share if we don't really know and that is frequently the case with young persons.

Families should be given an explanation of the success rate and complexity associated with resuscitation, but this should be presented in a sensitive way.[15,17,40,51] If families are told that resuscitation leads to breaking ribs and traumatic intubation, this might coerce the family into a do-not-resuscitate (DNR) order.[15] The attending neurologist should also explain the morbidity if the patient were to survive. This could then initiate a discussion about quality of life.[11,16,20,22,39] In this discussion, it is prudent to cover the possibility of depression, lack of focus and initiative, irritability, disinhibition, and the possibility of being wheelchair bound. Simple explanations such as "survive but handicapped," "survive but walk with a cane," "two-thirds will do poorly," or "cannot tell" are ambiguous and not helpful in explaining morbidity.[56] To state that a major brain injury with a handicap is worse than death is less than truthful and often not supported by studies that have examined patients surviving this injury.

A family conference should include summaries, and at multiple times, neurologists may ask the family for feedback. Families may be confused by what we mean by "comfort care" or "palliative care"; if it seems unclear, it could be explained that the aim of palliative care is to reduce suffering and promote comfort, resulting in a peaceful and natural death.[37]

In all prognostication discussions in the literature the term "self-fulfilling prophecy" has played an important role in defining the pitfalls of prognostication. Self-fulfilling prophecy is a concept that implies that outcome is a result of prediction. For example, an unwarranted pessimistic outlook on the patient's condition may lead to withdrawal of support or withdrawal of care and, therefore, a poor outcome. The thinking is that neurologists' predictions of poor outcome might contribute to mortality rates of patients with stroke, traumatic brain injury, and, in particular, anoxic-ischemic encephalopathy. Similarly, some would claim that an optimistic approach, in which all resuscitative measures are continued and aggressive care and going the extra mile are provided, could lead to improvement of the patient, but only if given the opportunity. The flip side of optimism may be false hope. Doing all that is medically possible may leave a person devastated and crippled and unable to experience even a reasonably good quality of life.

In any event, there is a true possible dualism. Optimistic and pessimistic attitudes—overall or specifically to the case—may result in a chain of decisions (Figure 8.1). Neurologists should also appreciate that during these conversations, an overly optimistic prognosis may be a symptom of a neurologist's emotional reaction to the clinical situation. On the other hand, a demoralized neurologist may be more willing to push families to proceed with withdrawal of care.[25,27,29,33]

No neurologist wants to deprive the patient or family of a possible good outcome or deprive them of hope, and the "self-fulfilling prophecy" has no role to play if the neurologist can prognosticate with a high degree of accuracy. Unfortunately, this is only possible in a few categories of patients—usually comatose patients with secondary brainstem injury unresponsive to aggressive measures.

The introduction of the concept of the self-fulfilling prophecy may lead to physicians feeling responsible for the death of their patients and can cause a fear of causing, or even hastening, death. The importance of the self-fulfilling prophecy can be exaggerated—that is, the concept is not applicable in all situations. For example, a patient who has lost almost all brainstem reflexes in the setting of a catastrophic brain injury is not expected to improve beyond a

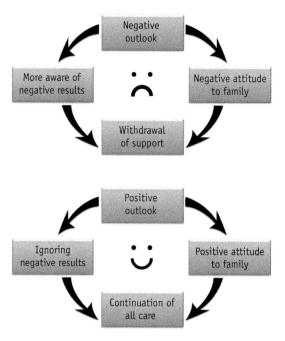

Figure 8.1 Consequences of a positive and negative attitude.

vegetative state; this is based on enormous empirical evidence. Withdrawal in that particular patient is based on good medical judgment and understanding of the neurobiological consequences of acute brain injury. Studies that evaluate prognostication will always be hampered by failing to measure factors that may make neurologists decide to withdraw support. This may be an intercurrent infection, a major complication requiring additional medical support, or certain neurologic findings that may not have been measured. For example, if all prognosis studies use only the Glasgow Coma Scale or an even less accurate definition of unconsciousness, important brainstem injury would not be taken into account and could significantly skew the data. Focusing too much on the possibility of a self-fulfilling prophecy logically leads in most cases to continuation of treatment and full resuscitative measures. It is not difficult to understand that some patients who have had a poor prognosis may ultimately have a poor outcome and that continuation of a high level of care would not serve any purpose.[12] On the other hand, to withdraw treatment in a patient who would have survived without any major impairment if full resuscitative measures had been continued simply shows poor judgment.

Withdrawal of support is a common cause of death in critically ill patients. Families may also decide to proceed with withdrawal of support in the setting of uncertainty. They may consider that the prospect of surviving as a severely disabled person, even if the chances are 50/50, might not be in their best interest and not commensurate with the patient's wishes. Staying on a ventilator, unable to return home, may not be the quality of life the patient desires.

In Practice

Patient-neurologist interaction consumes more time than analyzing, reviewing tests, and setting up a treatment plan. For many neurologists, their behavior is motivated by trying to be kind to the patient and family.[3] Neurologists understand that the important principle of autonomy may override any other principles. The patient has a choice. Neurologists may ask families what their understanding is of their loved one's illness. This will shape better understanding of care and also transitions in level of care. Uncertainty about prognosis is a given fact in many circumstances and acknowledgment of this uncertainty is helpful to families. Using uncertainty to postpone decisions may not be helpful and may be counterproductive.[46]

Neurologists should also identify special needs for family members in understanding their loved one's illness. Depression and anxiety should be recognized, not only in the patient but also in family members, particularly if patients have rapidly become gravely ill.[6,21,32] Neurologists need to recognize that in some families, lower levels of anxiety and depression are seen with higher levels of spiritual well-being. Neurologists may ask about sources of strength and comfort, and should ask patients if they are interested in speaking with a chaplain about their experiences. Chaplains provide spiritual care, usually regardless of patients' beliefs and practices. This is particularly important in certain regions of the United States. Given current globalization, religion plays an important role in discussions with family members. Theological discussions are outside the purview of the neurologist's experience and expertise, but a straightforward approach asking these simple questions may be very important and appreciated by the family.[1,23,35–38,49]

As mentioned before, the shared decision process is the current best approach to discuss level of care. Another often-used term is "substituted judgment," which de-links the family from decision-making and implies that it is not what the family wants nor what most people would want, but what the patient would say if he or she were able to voice his or her opinion. Neurologists should carefully explain to family members that they are not making decisions, but interpreting the loved one's values and preferences during a severe catastrophic illness.[13–15]

So how do these meetings progress logically, and what should be done? The meeting starts with introductions of the participants and explanation of the purpose and process of the meeting. Many family members need to understand that these meetings are simply to provide information and to explain the level of care, and that these meetings are not called specifically to discuss withdrawing of care.[9] As alluded to earlier, some neurologists do directly ask the family members what their understanding is of the illness of the patient; however, this requires considerable effort for some families and may be inappropriate in some situations. A better question is to ask them what their biggest concerns are and how they define good and bad case scenarios. If the family has a desire to speak, they should be allowed to vent their concerns, frustrations, and opinions without being interrupted.[18]

Ethnicity and socioeconomic status impact conversations and the words we use.[31] This may have to do with cultural communication styles or cultural preferences regarding end-of-life care. It is important to ask whether the family feels that the patient is suffering and whether they are certain the patient is comfortable and in no distress. It may not be useful to discuss how their loved one has responded to acute illness in the past. This may not be relevant, because the current illness may be obviously far more severe and likely different. Families often bring out prior experiences when their loved one has been involved in situations with other family members. The family may recall conversations when the patient clearly discussed what is acceptable and unacceptable, but the specificity of these statements always remains difficult to judge. Many families would say that they do not want the patient to "be a vegetable" or "like the Schiavo case" or "plugged to a wall." Sometimes the fear that improvement would lead to the patient being more aware of future major disability may play a role. For many families it is not justified to continue care if there is a high likelihood of loss of independence and of the things that make life so enjoyable.

The most important task is to explain the clinical situation and the state of the patient. It should be clear to family members that neurologists are taking all measures to relieve suffering. Prognostication should be discussed via a qualitative statement or a numerical statement. An example of a qualitative statement is "I think the patient will remain disabled and will most likely die after we withdraw support." An example of a numerical statement is, for example, "80% of patients in this situation do not survive." Both these approaches can be used in disclosing the news of a poor prognosis.[24] Many families understand that a perfect prediction is difficult and in some instances as poor as a seismologist predicting a major earthquake when there are already rumblings (it is only 5% likely). When discussing resuscitation status, one should avoid the words "withdrawing of care" and should emphasize that everything is being done for the patient.[2,43–45]

During these conversations, families will grieve and cry. It is a common observation, however, that after the family has made a decision to withdraw care, the mood often changes for the good and that families come to terms rather quickly and stabilize in their relationships. Sadness often quickly turns to relief (and even laughter). A follow-up meeting is necessary and should be planned. This can be the next day, or later in the day, when other family members have arrived, or when family members have had the opportunity to discuss the situation in detail.[50,54]

The most important need at the end of life is to be treated as a whole person and to maintain one's dignity. Not dying alone—but in the presence of close friends—must be important.[47]

By the Way

- Avoid empty phrases, triteness and stereotypes
- If there is no way to tell, let family know there is no way to tell
- Availability and responsiveness is key
- Communicate with nursing staff and family as frequently as possible, not just during rounds
- Undivided attention to families' concerns is necessary

Neurologic Outcome by the Numbers

- ~60% of patients of all ages survive in-hospital resuscitation
- ~40% of comatose patients may die in first two weeks of hospitalization
- ~20% of patients with severe brain injury get an early DNR order
- ~10% of patients with acute brain injury may be able to donate organs
- ~1% of patients with deteriorating acute brain injury survive CPR

Putting It All Together

- Appreciate that conversations with families require a separate place and the opportunity to speak to all involved
- The important components that make up compassion are honesty, accountability and authenticity
- Optimism and pessimism have no role in straightforward conversations
- Whether the patient may achieve autonomy and dignity determines the level of care

References

1. Al-Yousefi NA. Observations of Muslim neurologists regarding the influence of religion on health and their clinical approach. *J Relig Health* 2012;51:269–280.

2. Anderson WG, Chase R, Pantilat SZ, Tulsky JA, Auerbach AD. Code status discussions between attending hospitalist neurologists and medical patients at hospital admission. *J Gen Intern Med* 2011;26:359–366.

3. Armstrong J. Fellow suffering. *J Clin Oncol* 2004;22:4425–4427.

4. Asch DA, Shea JA, Jedrziewski MK, et al. The limits of suffering: critical care nurses' views of hospital care at the end of life. *Soc Sci Med* 1997;45:1661–1668.

5. Ausman JI. Trust, malpractice, and honesty in medicine: should doctors say they are sorry? *Surg Neurol* 2006;66:105–106.

6. Azoulay E, Pochard F, Kentish-Barnes N, et al. Risk of post-traumatic stress symptoms in family members of intensive care unit patients. *Am J Respir Crit Care Med* 2005;171: 987–994.

7. Bernat JL. Ethical aspects of determining and communicating prognosis in critical care. *Neurocrit Care* 2004;1:107–117.

8. Billings JA. The end-of-life family meeting in intensive care. Part II. Family-centered decision making. *J Palliat Med* 2011;14:1051–1057.

9. Billings JA, Block SD. The end-of-life family meeting in intensive care. Part III. A guide for structured discussions. *J Palliat Med* 2011;14:1058–1064.

10. Boehm FH. Teaching bedside manners to medical students. *Acad Med* 2008;83:534.

11. Burns JP, Edwards J, Johnson J, Cassem NH, Truog RD. Do-not-resuscitate order after 25 years. *Crit Care Med* 2003;31:1543–1550.

12. Burns JP, Truog RD. Futility: a concept in evolution. *Chest* 2007;132:1987–1993.

13. Curtis JR, Engelberg RA, Wenrich MD, et al. Studying communication about end-of-life care during the ICU family conference: development of a framework. *J Crit Care* 2002;17:147–160.

14. Curtis JR, Engelberg RA, Wenrich MD, et al. Missed opportunities during family conferences about end-of-life care in the intensive care unit. *Am J Respir Crit Care Med* 2005;171: 844–849.

15. Curtis JR, Park DR, Krone MR, Pearlman RA. Use of the medical futility rationale in do-not-attempt-resuscitation orders. *JAMA* 1995;273:124–128.

16. Downar J, Hawryluck L. What should we say when discussing "code status" and life support with a patient? A Delphi analysis. *J Palliat Med* 2010;13:185–195.

17. Flamm AL. The Texas "futility" procedure: no such thing as a fairy-tale ending. *Med Ethics* 2004;11:4–11.

18. Francis LK. Learning to listen: a fellow's experience. *J Clin Oncol* 2006;24:3209–3210.

19. Fried TR, Bradley EH, O'Leary J. Changes in prognostic awareness among seriously ill older persons and their caregivers. *Palliat Med* 2006;9:61–69.

20. Hofmann JC, Wenger NS, Davis RB, et al. Patient preferences for communication with neurologists about end-of-life decisions: SUPPORT Investigators: Study to Understand Prognoses and Preference for Outcomes and Risks of Treatment. *Ann Intern Med* 1997;127:1–12.

21. Johnson KS, Tulsky JA, Hays JC, et al. Which domains of spirituality are associated with anxiety and depression in patients with advanced illness? *J Gen Intern Med* 2011;26:751–758.

22. Klaristenfeld DD, Harrington DT, Miner TJ. Teaching palliative care and end-of-life issues: a core curriculum for surgical residents. *Ann Surg Oncol* 2007;14:1801–1806.

23. Kuczewski MG. Talking about spirituality in the clinical setting: can being professional require being personal? *Am J Bioeth* 2007;7:4–11.

24. Lee Char SJ, Evans LR, Malvar GL, White DB. A randomized trial of two methods to disclose prognosis to surrogate decision makers in intensive care units. *Am J Respir Crit Care Med* 2010;182:905–909.

25. Levin TT, Moreno B, Silvester W, Kissane DW. End-of-life communication in the intensive care unit. *Gen Hosp Psychiatry* 2010;32:433–442.

26. Liben S. Words matter: the importance of the language we use. *J Palliat Med* 2011;14:128.

27. Lilly CM, De Meo DL, Sonna LA, et al. An intensive communication intervention for the critically ill. *Am J Med* 2000;109:469–475.

28. Loprinzi CL, Schapira L, Moynihan T, et al. Compassionate honesty. *J Palliat Med* 2010;13:1187–1191.

29. Meltzer LS, Huckabay LM. Critical care nurses' perceptions of futile care and its effect on burnout. *Am J Crit Care* 2004;13:202–208.

30. Morris DA, Johnson KS, Ammarell N, et al. What is your understanding of your illness? A communication tool to explore patients' perspectives of living with advanced illness. *J Gen Intern Med* 2012;27:1460–1466.

31. Muni S, Engelberg RA, Treece PD, Dotolo D, Curtis JR. The influence of race/ethnicity and socioeconomic status on end-of-life care in the ICU. *Chest* 2011;139:1025–1033.

32. Noorani NH, Montagnini M. Recognizing depression in palliative care patients. *J Palliat Med* 2007;10:458–464.

33. Norris K, Merriman MP, Curtis JR, et al. Next of kin perspectives on the experience of end-of-life care in the community setting. *J Palliat Med* 2007;10:1101–1105.

34. Owen D, Davidson J. Hubris syndrome: an acquired personality disorder? A study of US Presidents and UK Prime Ministers over the last 100 years. *Brain* 2009;132:1396–1406.

35. Oyama O, Koenig HG. Religious beliefs and practices in family medicine. *Arch Fam Med* 1998;7:431–435.

36. Phelps AC, Lauderdale KE, Alcorn S, et al. Addressing spirituality within the care of patients at the end of life: perspectives of patients with advanced cancer, oncologists, and oncology nurses. *J Clin Oncol* 2012;30:2538–2544.

37. Puchalski CM, Larson DB. Developing curricula in spirituality and medicine. *Acad Med* 1998;73:970–974.

38. Puchalski C, Romer AL. Taking a spiritual history allows clinicians to understand patients more fully. *J Palliat Med* 2000;3:129–137.

39. Rabinstein AA. Ethical dilemmas in the neurologic ICU: withdrawing life-support measures after devastating brain injury. *Continuum* 2009;15:13–25.

40. Rabinstein AA, McClelland RL, Wijdicks EFM, Manno EM, Atkinson JL. Cardiopulmonary resuscitation in critically ill neurologic-neurosurgical patients. *Mayo Clin Proc* 2004;79:1391–1395.

41. Rodin G, Mackay JA, Zimmermann C, et al. Clinician-patient communication: a systematic review. *Support Care Cancer* 2009;17:627–644.

42. Salerno JA. Restoring trust through bioethics education? *Acad Med* 2008;83:532–534.

43. Schneiderman LJ, Gilmer T, Teetzel HD. Impact of ethics consultations in the intensive care setting: a randomized, controlled trial. *Crit Care Med* 2000;28:3920–3924.

44. Selph RB, Shiang J, Engelberg R, Curtis JR, White DB. Empathy and life support decisions in intensive care units. *J Gen Intern Med* 2008;23:1311–1317.

45. Shanawani H, Wenrich MD, Tonelli MR, Curtis JR. Meeting neurologists' responsibilities in providing end-of-life care. *Chest* 2008;133:775–786.

46. Smith AK, White DB, Arnold RM. Uncertainty—the other side of prognosis. *N Engl J Med* 2013;368:2448–2450.

47. Steinhauser KE, Arnold RM, Olsen MK, et al. Comparing three life-limiting diseases: does diagnosis matter or is sick, sick? *J Pain Symptom Manage* 2011;42:331–341.

48. Steinhauser KE, Christakis NA, Clipp EC, et al. Factors considered important at the end of life by patients, family, neurologists, and other care providers. *JAMA* 2000;284:2476–2482.

49. Steinhauser KE, Voils CI, Clipp EC, et al. "Are you at peace?": one item to probe spiritual concerns at the end of life. *Arch Intern Med* 2006;166:101–105.

50. Sullivan AM, Lakoma MD, Billings JA, et al. Teaching and learning end-of-life care: evaluation of a faculty development program in palliative care. *Acad Med* 2005;80:657–668.

51. Tian J, Kaufman DA, Zarich S, et al. Outcomes of critically ill patients who received cardio-pulmonary resuscitation. *Am J Respir Crit Care Med* 2010;182:501–506.

52. Treadway K, Chatterjee N. Into the water: the clinical clerkships. *N Engl J Med* 2011;364:1190–1193.

53. Truog RD. Patients and doctors: evolution of a relationship. *N Engl J Med* 2012;366:581–585.

54. Weissman DE. Decision making at a time of crisis near the end of life. *JAMA* 2004;292: 1738–1743.

55. White DB, Braddock CH 3rd, Bereknyei S, Curtis JR. Toward shared decision making at the end of life in intensive care units: opportunities for improvement. *Arch Intern Med* 2007;167:461–467.

56. Wijdicks EFM, Rabinstein AA. Absolutely no hope? Some ambiguity of futility of care in devastating acute stroke. *Crit Care Med* 2004;32:2332–2342.

57. Wijdicks EFM, Rabinstein AA. The family conference: end-of-life guidelines at work for comatose patients. *Neurology* 2007;68:1092–1094.

9

Withdrawal of Support and Palliation

Withdrawal of support and palliation is an accepted—and often very appropriate—decision at the end of life. It encompasses decisions to withhold resuscitation attempts, to remove the mechanical ventilator and extubate the patient, or to stop the administration of drugs that serve no purpose. These decisions should be based on extensive medical information. They can be made almost immediately when an unsurvivable catastrophic neurologic illness occurs in a patient with previously expressed wishes.[14]

But far more commonly, the issue of why aggressive care is continued comes up after a prolonged illness and multiple attempts at treating the disorder (e.g., refractory status epilepticus or failure to improve from a major stroke). Most patients with acute neurologic disease can potentially survive and mortality is linked to withdrawal (or withholding) of care. However, it would be disingenuous to state that death in a neurologic patient is caused by withdrawal of care, because the truth of the matter is that support simply interrupted the natural dying sequence.

As discussed in more detail in Chapters 7 and 8, these decisions may be guided by strong personal views and may be influenced by cultural, religious, and other social factors.[13,17,23] Even a personal situation (at least in the United States), such as inability to financially support long-term care in a patient, may play an important role in how decisions are made particularly in families under duress.

When decisions on withdrawal of care are made, how do we interpret advance directives? How do we best provide comfort to the patient and family? What are the most important medical issues and logistics to attend to? This chapter discusses some of the principles to adequately provide palliation. There are several society and council recommendations based on consensus opinion.[10,12,23]

Principles

In the discussion on withdrawal of support, families should be provided options and a direction. The options are types of withdrawal—extubation, discontinuation of all medication, do-not-resuscitate (DNR) orders—usually in some sort of combination, stepwise, or all at once. The direction—a peaceful dying process—should be explained to the family members to a certain degree so that they can reasonably anticipate what will happen. Withdrawal of support implies no hydration or feeding, and families should be told that this does not lead to discomfort to the patient (it is not an agonizing hunger strike). Some estimate of time to cardiac arrest should be provided based on clinical examination, but noting that if the patient does not die within hours, it may take several days or even 2 weeks. It largely depends on the patient's state of hydration and current kidney function.[5]

Advance directives, used in many countries, are legal documents in which the patient has determined what actions should be taken if no longer able to make decisions due to illness or incapacity. The documents can come in many forms: some simply designate that a person with power of attorney may make decisions about the patient; others, such as a living will, leave instructions for treatment and are more detailed and specific. Usually these advance directives specify when there is care in a terminal condition, and these living wills have been clearly written in order not to prolong care in the setting of futility. Physicians cannot ignore advance directives and just claim to be acting in good faith and in accordance with good professional practice. Directives need to be followed whenever available.

Three types of directives are known.

- A *living will* gives specific direction on healthcare or appoints an agent or proxy to make decisions on the patient's behalf when there is a serious or terminal illness. It should, in broad terms, instruct surrogate decision-makers whether to withhold or withdraw treatment in dire situations and at the end of life.
- *Durable power of attorney for healthcare* authorizes another person (agent or proxy) to make decisions on the patient's behalf even though the patient may not be terminally ill.
- A *mental health declaration* provides specific direction or designates a proxy to make decisions about intrusive mental health treatment (e.g., electroshock therapy and neuroleptic medications).

Generally, there is a low rate of completion of advance directives and it remains uncertain whether education and promotion may increase the number of patients with advance directives. Therefore, in reality, currently decision-making in most situations will not involve an advance directive. The questions asked of family members should involve assessment of burdens the patient would not be able to bear. Family members would have to decide on that unanimously and in cases involving elderly patients, often the children are best positioned to assess that.

Many states in the United States offer the possibility of obtaining a living will. Most living wills have general statements that make it abundantly obvious that if struck by an illness with no hope in sight, the signer of the document would want to forgo any extraordinary measures. Some living wills specifically direct when to stop resuscitation using a time limit (e.g., no longer than 30 minutes); others mention time on the mechanical ventilation ("only short term") or request only oxygen mask or noninvasive breathing support such as biphasic positive airway pressure (BiPAP). Each of these amendments potentially increases ambiguity and further uncertainty with family members. In these documents, the definition of care beyond cardiopulmonary resuscitation is often inadequate to guide therapy, and discussions with the family and occasionally with patients are needed for clarification. Only a minority of advance directives may include clear statements on cardiopulmonary resuscitation, mechanical ventilation, defibrillation, nutritional assistance, (parenteral or enteral) DNR, blood transfusion or plasma expanders. A order specifies no resuscitation in the event of cardiac or respiratory arrest but may also include no intravenous drugs for acute cardiac arrhythmias, invasive monitoring devices, hemodialysis, cardiac pacemakers, endotracheal tubes, chest tubes, cardioversion, or bronchoscopy. Although many US states recognize advance directives from other states, some do not. Physicians should know the laws in their state of practice.

A DNR order is part of a decision that can be driven by a living will. When to address these DNR orders is unclear; however, most hospitals advise that resuscitation orders be addressed on admission. Families typically first will request full code, but ask for a DNR status after noticing no progress in care. DNR may be considered if there simply is a clinical situation that is overwhelmingly bad. It is an important ethical principle for physicians not to allow their personal biases to influence these decisions, and that may go both ways. Families understand that the decision to make a DNR order is based on the best medical information. This relieves the family of the burden to take a major role in these decisions.

Patients have the right to discontinue any type of medical intervention, including mechanical ventilation or even noninvasive assisted ventilation, at any time they wish, even if they know it would lead to death. This is separate from a refusal of medical intervention and also separate from assistance with dying.

Withholding therapy means avoidance of resuscitative measures, which can include dialysis, placement of tracheostomy or gastrostomy, antibiotics for ongoing infection, vasopressors or isotopes, and insulin infusion. Many European countries have opted for withholding care rather than a sudden transition to palliative care.

Sedation orders are commonplace after extubation of the patient with evidence of responsiveness to the environment. These are patients with stupor but also may be more alert patients with a locked-in syndrome, end-stage amyotrophic lateral sclerosis (ALS), or cervical cord transection. Knowledge of the details of palliative sedation orders are imperative to assure the care is being provided.

A major bioethical topic is the principle of double effect of sedation. This philosophical term (with roots in catholic thought) implies that administration of a potent sedative (or anesthetic) results in relief of distress (its intended primary effect) but also in the possibility of hastening death (side effect) due to inability to adequately breathe or maintain an airway while "heavily" sedated. Recently it has been explained as "good" and "bad" effects. A good effect would be "morally good"; a bad effect would be not specifically intended but expected and unavoidable. The administration of a sedative drug requires that "the good outweighs the bad," and a "good effect" cannot come from a bad action such as administration of a neuromuscular blocker with potassium chloride (essentially euthanasia).[21]

Sedatives should be administered anticipatorily to achieve a rapid effect (arbitrarily defined as a calm, drowsy, nonanxious, or nonagitated patient).[7] Orders should be as the circumstances require rather than automatically escalating. Rapid increase in the dose without a documented reason could potentially cause questioning of intent—in legal proceedings it could be challenged by family members.

Some have suggested a preemptive high dose of sedatives and opioids before extubation, but this practice is not encouraged. Some families may sense they are simply participating in euthanasia if the patient dies very quickly.[2,20]

After the decision has been made to provide palliative measures only every physician should keep possible organ or tissue donation in mind. No organ donation agency should be formally contacted (or speak with the family members) until the decision to withdraw support has been made. Failure to prevent this may lead to unnecessary suspicion that withdrawal of support is intended to facilitate organ donation. When the decision is made to withdraw support, donation after cardiac death (DCD) can be requested. This is typically in patients who are less than 60 years old and have suitable organs for donation. Donation after cardiac circulatory death is widely accepted and used in many countries.

In Practice

End-of-life practices vary by country and are best known in Europe and the United States.[8,11,18,23,24,25] End-of-life practices are common in European intensive care units (ICUs) but the choice to limit life-sustaining therapy was related to age, type of diagnosis, number of days in the ICU, availability of an intensivist, and physician religion.[1,17] In the United States, similar factors play a role but also racial differences.[16]

Withdrawal of life-support measures consists of extubation and discontinuation of any administered drugs. Central access and arterial catheters are removed.

Transport to a single quiet room—in the event the patient remains stable—is reasonable after a certain amount of time has passed.

There are other important nursing care issues. All unnecessary equipment should be removed, and the monitor in the room is disconnected (while other monitors of the patient can still be used). Noise and light should be minimized. Chairs for family members should be available. Physicians can be very helpful in support by being present and should be silent and respectful.

The use of opioids and sedatives during withdrawal of mechanical ventilation is variable and dependent on patients being comatose.[3,4,6] Usually midazolam, propofol, or fentanyl are used in a low dose to provide comfort to the patient. Withdrawal of care also involves discontinuation of nutrition and hydration, extubation, discontinuation of supportive pharmaceutical agents, and administration of fentanyl or lorazepam if the patient develops labored breathing or shows significant unrest. This is far less common in patients with acute neurologic disease, and these measures are typically not necessary if the patient is comatose. Rapidly escalating the dose after extubation is problematic, although there is no evidence that it could hasten death. Options such as a dose of fentanyl less than 100 mcg/h, morphine less than 25 mg/h, midazolam less than 10 mg/h, propofol less than 50 mg/h, and lorazepam fusion less than 0.3 mg/h are acceptable amounts before and after withdrawal of mechanical ventilation. Terminal sedation ought to be permissible and part of palliation, and the administration of opiates for palliation is ethical and legal in all US states.

In our institution, it is common practice to start a morphine infusion of 0.1 mg/kg/h and titrate to comfort by increasing infusion with small increments every 15 minutes. In addition, we may institute a lorazepam infusion of 0.05 mg/kg/h and titrate upward slowly until symptoms of agitation or restlessness are controlled. In deeply comatose patients, none of this is indicated unless breathing after extubation becomes markedly labored. Most patients with secondary brainstem injury die within hours after life support is withdrawn.

After removal of the endotracheal tube, the patient may breathe or not. Most emotional responses of the family members are around that time quickly making way for acceptance.

The patient should be positioned so as to facilitate airflow and frequent suctioning may be needed. Breathing may be noisy and rattling and a source of distress for families.[9,10] Such breathing is often called agonal (a term that, when used in conversation, often is misinterpreted as indicating agony of the patient). When a change in head and body position is unsuccessful, glycopyrrolate or subcutaneous scopolamine or a patch can be used. Scopolamine relaxes the smooth muscles, and both drugs dry up the secretions. Terminal dry mouth is managed with oral hygiene every 2–4 hours, smoothing the lips with Vaseline, and moist air. Terminal vomiting from increased intracranial pressure can be treated with

25–50 mg of promethazine rectally, metoclopramide, haloperidol, or ondanse-tron, 32 mg intravenously but this is very uncommon. Hiccups can be relieved with baclofen (10 mg oral dose) before withdrawal of the gastrointestinal tube. Extreme agitation may be treated with 2 mg of lorazepam intravenously or, if necessary, midazolam, or propofol infusion.

Seizures may reoccur in patients when antiepileptic drugs are discontinued, but this possibility can be anticipated by administering midazolam intramuscu-larly before extubation. The family should be told that this drug is now used for careful palliation. Vigorous myoclonus status epilepticus may be very distressful to family members. Because we have not been successful with any of the anti-epileptic drugs, one option is to proceed with propofol infusion for several hours, discontinue it, and then withdraw support.

Several acute neurologic disorders pose major management problems. Not uncommonly, ALS is diagnosed in ICUs when patients are admitted with respi-ratory distress and in retrospect, have had a history of progressive generalized weakness. The preferences toward withdrawal of care are usually not known. Some patients want to live as long as possible, and many claim a good quality of life.

Not all patients with advanced ALS are aware that respiratory failure is likely to develop, and fewer than half have discussed this problem with their physician. Very few make their decision before the emergence of respiratory failure, even when they have suffered with the disorder for many months. Many intensivists have had the experience with a patient with ALS triaged to the ICU but with no prior family discussion or family understanding of the severity of the illness. Physicians have a major responsibility to discuss the illness and its expectant prognosis, but unfortunately some again postpone or avoid any discussion.

In deciding whether to withdraw support in ALS, it is important to exclude intermittent pulmonary infections or other disorders that may contribute to the patient's state. When a patient decides to discontinue ventilation, removal of the ventilator may be very uncomfortable to the patient and cause immediate air hunger. Slow weaning with supplemental oxygen produces further retention of carbon dioxide and eventually coma. Slow weaning can be performed in sequen-tial steps with evaluation of the patient after each step. First, FiO_2 is reduced to room air and positive end-expiratory pressure (PEEP) is reduced to zero. If this leads to discomfort, sedation may be titrated upward. This is then followed by weaning intermittent mandatory ventilation (IMV) to pressure support, and its effect is assessed for at least 1 hour. If the patient—with sedation—is comfort-able at IMV of 4 and on a pressure support of 5 cm water (closely similar to spon-taneous breathing), the patient is placed on a T-piece or extubated. This method seems preferable, coupled with several doses of morphine to counter possible sig-naled discomfort.

Another major problem is sudden devastating traumatic quadriplegia. Complete cervical transection with apnea usually precludes recovery, but 28%–57% of the patients with injuries at the C3 level or lower may recover. The ethical questions in patients with traumatic quadriplegia and ventilator dependency are very difficult. It is unusual for a patient with full knowledge of the consequences to ask emphatically to have the ventilator removed. In follow-up interviews at rehabilitation centers, assessments were predominantly positive, with up to 93% of the patients "glad to be alive." Although many patients express some degree of hopelessness and despondency, many also change their mind with the passage of time.

When requests to turn off the ventilator continue evaluation by an ethics committee, is required whether to honor the request. It is difficult to judge whether the patient's request is a rational choice and whether the patient is capable of autonomous choice. The patient should be presented with all relevant facts and rehabilitation options. Postponing the decision is wise, but some patients with a complete transection may continue to forcefully reject any such suggestion. The ventilator can be withdrawn if the patient refuses to reconsider, because any patient may exercise the right to refuse life-sustaining treatment. These decisions can be very stressful to caregivers who may disagree with the decision.

Withdrawal of support in a patient with a locked-in syndrome due to a basilar artery thrombus is equally difficult. Unfortunately (or fortunately), level of consciousness varies, and early on in the clinical course it is difficult to establish a reliable communication with the patient. Moreover, patients with more function than a typical locked-in syndrome may improve further in the ensuing months, even to a point of independence. The decisions here are based on certainty of a permanent deficit and prior wishes of the patient. The withdrawal sequence should be similar to that of a patient with a spinal cord injury.

Withdrawal of support in a patient with a catastrophic, irreversible brain injury may involve patients who fulfill the clinical criteria of brain death or patients who still have retained brainstem function. In patients who fulfill the clinical criteria of brain death, the first line of action is to have family discuss possible organ donation with a representative of an organ donation agency. Most families agree with organ donation but if the family still refuses organ donation after detailed explanation, if there has been previous documentation that the patient would not want to be an organ donor, or if the patient is not suitable for organ donation or tissue harvesting, care can be withdrawn and cardiac arrest will occur in approximately 5–10 minutes as a result of rapid desaturation due to apnea. The family can be at the bedside, although brief twitching extremities can occur as a result of rapidly induced hypoxemia of the spinal cord. In many instances, the patient remains immobile, will become cyanotic, and death can be declared after circulation stops.

In patients with a catastrophic injury who do have a severe brainstem injury and when there is consensus about the irreversibility of this condition, withdrawal of support will often also lead to cardiopulmonary arrest. Of all patients with a catastrophic injury, approximately half die within one hour of withdrawal of support; the other half may take a day or even several days. For several reasons, it might be useful to know how long the dying process will take. We have developed a prediction scale, shown in Figure 9.1, that accurately predicts death within 1 hour.[15] Taking into account the corneal reflexes no (absent one point), cough reflex (absent two points), absent motor response or extensor responses (one point), or an increased oxygenation index calculated as $100 \times$ ($FiO_2 \times$ mean airway pressure in cm water divided by PaO_2 in mm Hg; one point when more than 3). If all of these components are present (sum score of 5), less than 10% of the patients will survive beyond 1 hour.

This is also important information when planning donation after cardiac death (DCD). Whether the patients are eligible is determined after careful evaluation by an organ procurement coordinator and this is a time-consuming process. The patient is transferred to the operating room and prepared and draped for organ retrieval. After extubation, circulatory arrest is determined and usually involves palpating the carotid artery, auscultation of the heart, and documentation of absent reading of the arterial line. After circulatory arrest is determined, 5 minutes of additional waiting are mandated before the surgical team proceeds with organ retrieval (in several European countries 10 minutes). Moreover, families are allowed— if they choose—to be in the operating room until circulatory arrest and are led away before the 5 minutes "death watch". This procedure is different in patients who have been declared brain dead, in which case surgeons proceed immediately with retrieval of organs, often while there is still adequate circulation.

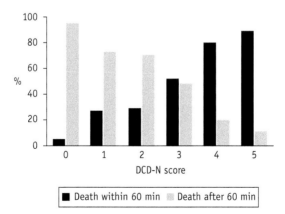

Figure 9.1 Probability of death after withdrawal of support (N-DCD scale). (From reference 15)

The determination of brain death is relatively uncommon and occurs in only 10% of all patients with a catastrophic neurologic injury. The basis of brain death determination is predicated on the documentation of irreversible coma of which the cause is known, neuroimaging that explains coma, absent sedative or paralytic drugs, absence of severe acid–base electrolyte or endocrine abnormality, a normal or near-normal temperature, absence of shock defined as a systolic blood pressure <100 mm Hg, and no spontaneous respiration. Brain death examination includes testing of pupil reflexes to light, corneal reflexes to touch, eye motility, facial movements to noxious stimuli, gag reflex, cough reflex, motor response to noxious stimuli, and an apnea test. The apnea test is typically performed using the oxygen diffusion method, in which the patient is preoxygenated with 100% FiO_2 for 10 minutes, the ventilator is disconnected, and oxygen is administered via an insufflation catheter to the level of the carina. When there is no breathing effort arterial blood gases are drawn at 8–10 minutes while the patient remains disconnected from the ventilator. A PCO_2 of ≥60 mm Hg or 20 mm Hg rise from normal baseline PCO_2 value is considered a sufficient stimulus of the respiratory centers. After this blood gas determination the patient is reconnected to the ventilator. These examinations will confirm absence of brain stem function. Brain death can be declared with one examination in most US states. A second examination is required in eight US states (Alaska, California, Connecticut, Florida, Iowa, Kentucky, Louisiana, Virginia). After brain death declaration, either a patient becomes an organ donor or care is withdrawn. In extreme circumstances, the family may want to continue ventilatory and circulatory support (this quandary is discussed further in Chapter 10).

By the Way

- The patient is usually undisturbed by noisy terminal respirations
- Parenteral fluids may cause patient's discomfort due to increased body water, gastric and pulmonary secretions
- Use multipurpose drugs to treat anxiety and pain
- Nebulized furosemide may help in dyspnea
- High fever requires treatment with cooling blankets

Neuropalliation by the Numbers

- ~90% of pain in terminally ill patients can be relieved
- ~80% of patients' infusion rate of analgesics does not change in the final hours
- ~50% of patients with a neurocatastrophy die in one hour after extubation
- ~10% of patients with neurocatastrophy and normal brainstem reflexes die one hour after extubation
- ~5% of patients develop seizures after discontinuation of antiepileptics

---

Putting It All Together

- Patients have the right to discontinue any type of medical intervention
- Neuropalliation is different from palliative care
- Midazolam, propofol, or fentanyl can be used in a low dose to provide comfort to the patient
- Withdrawal of support from a comatose patient does not require palliative measures such as sedation or pain medication
- Probability of death after withdrawal of support after a neurocatastrophy can be calculated

References

1. Azoulay E, Metnitz B, Sprung CL, et al. End-of-life practices in 282 intensive care units: data from the SAPS 3 database. *Intensive Care Medicine* 2009;35:623–630.
2. Billings JA. Humane terminal extubation reconsidered: the role for preemptive analgesia and sedation. *Crit Care Med* 2012;40:625–630.
3. Campbell ML. How to withdraw mechanical ventilation: a systematic review of the literature. *AACN Adv Crit Care* 2007;18:397–403.
4. Epker JL, Bakker J, Kompanje EJ. The use of opioids and sedatives and time until death after withdrawing mechanical ventilation and vasoactive drugs in a Dutch intensive care unit. *Anesth Analg* 2011;112:628–634.
5. Gerstel E, Engelberg RA, Koepsell T, Curtis JR. Duration of withdrawal of life support in the intensive care unit and association with family satisfaction. *Am J Respir Crit Care Med* 2008;178:798–804.
6. Hall RI, Rocker GM. End-of-life care in the ICU: treatments provided when life support was or was not withdrawn. *Chest* 2000;118:1424–1430.
7. Hawryluck LA, Harvey WR, Lemieux-Charles L, Singer PA. Consensus guidelines on analgesia and sedation in dying intensive care unit patients. *BMC Med Ethics* 2002;3:E3.
8. Keenan SP, Busche KD, Chen LM, et al. A retrospective review of a large cohort of patients undergoing the process of withholding or withdrawal of life support. *Crit Care Med* 1997;25:1324–1331.

9. Kompanje EJ, van der Hoven B, Bakker J. Anticipation of distress after discontinuation of mechanical ventilation in the ICU at the end of life. *Intensive Care Med* 2008;34:1593–1599.

10. Lanken PN, Terry PB, Delisser HM, et al. An official American Thoracic Society clinical policy statement: palliative care for patients with respiratory diseases and critical illnesses. *Am J Respir Crit Care Med* 2008;177:912–927.

11. Lee DK, Swinburne AJ, Fedullo AJ, Wahl GW. Withdrawing care: experience in a medical intensive care unit. *JAMA* 1994;271:1358–1361.

12. Lippert FK, Raffay V, Georgiou M, Steen PA, Bossaert L. European Resuscitation Council Guidelines for Resuscitation 2010. Section 10. The ethics of resuscitation and end-of-life decisions. *Resuscitation* 2010;81:1445–1451.

13. Mehta S. The intensive care unit continuum of care: easing death. *Crit Care Med* 2012;40: 700–701.

14. Prendergast TJ, Claessens MT, Luce JM. A national survey of end-of-life care for critically ill patients. *Am J Respir Crit Care Med* 1998;158:1163–1167.

15. Rabinstein AA, Yee AH, Mandrekar J, et al. Prediction of potential for organ donation after cardiac death in patients in neurocritical state: a prospective observational study. *Lancet Neurol* 2012;11:414–419.

16. Rubin MA, Dhar R, and Diringer MN. Racial differences in withdrawal of mechanical ventilation do not alter mortality in neurologically injured patients. *J Crit Care* 2014;29:44–53.

17. Sprung CL, Cohen SL, Sjokvist P, et al. End-of-life practices in European intensive care units: the Ethicus Study. *JAMA* 2003;290:790–797.

18. Teres D. Trends from the United States with end of life decisions in the intensive care unit. *Intensive Care Med* 1993;19:316–322.

19. Toossi S, Lomen-Hoerth C, Josephson SA, et al. Organ donation after cardiac death in amyotrophic lateral sclerosis. *Ann Neurol* 2012;71:154–156.

20. Treece PD, Engelberg RA, Crowley L, et al. Evaluation of a standardized order form for the withdrawal of life support in the intensive care unit. *Crit Care Med* 2004;32:1141–1148.

21. Truog RD, Brock DW, White DB. Should patients receive general anesthesia prior to extubation at the end of life? *Crit Care Med* 2012;40:631–633.

22. Truog RD, Burns JP, Mitchell C, Johnson J, Robinson W. Pharmacologic paralysis and withdrawal of mechanical ventilation at the end of life. *N Engl J Med* 2000;342:508–511.

23. Truog RD, Cist AF, Brackett SE, et al. Recommendations for end-of-life care in the intensive care unit: The Ethics Committee of the Society of Critical Care Medicine. *Crit Care Med* 2001;29:2332–2348.

24. Vincent JL, Parquier JN, Preiser JC, Brimioulle S, Kahn RJ. Terminal events in the intensive care unit: review of 258 fatal cases in one year. *Crit Care Med* 1989;17:530–533.

25. Wunsch H, Harrison DA, Harvey S, Rowan K. End-of-life decisions: a cohort study of the withdrawal of all active treatment in intensive care units in the United Kingdom. *Intensive Care Med* 2005;31:823–831.

10

Troubleshooting: Families Who
Won't Let Go

When they die nearly all patients in hospitals do after discontinuation of treatment—some after unsuccessful resuscitation, some with no medical intervention at all. Withdrawal of support or withdrawal of resuscitative measures in hopelessly sick patients is a common and, in the eyes of many of us, entirely appropriate measure. These decisions are made after meetings with family members and after a consensus is reached that further treatment is meaningless. A carefully executed conference will be reconciliatory in the overwhelming proportion of cases. Contacts with families are nearly always pleasant and cordial, leading to decisions by consensus.[2]

However, there are patients—and, in acute neurology, more often families—who want to pursue any option and believe that withholding intensive care is a poor decision no matter what. In their mind, every individual should be given the maximal chance.

End-of-life care has become politicized. End-of-life care—in the United States—has been associated with so-called death panels—reflecting a mistaken concern about a hypothetical rationing board denying expensive lifesaving care to contain costs. Some family members reason that even if physicians say that "there is nothing that can be done," it is basically untrue, and that many complications, including serious ones, can potentially be treated to sustain life with some quality.[17]

Approaching families who hope for a miraculously good outcome in a grave situation is common and always will be. The potential for later guilt over "doing something you may have to live with the rest of your life" may play a role.

Severe irreversible brain injury cannot be treated— in these cases, all interventions are ineffectual. Given all this, why do families not see the reality of the situation and why can they not come to terms? Why do families believe physicians are inaccurate in prediction? What are the main mechanisms that drive this failure to arrive at a mutual conclusion? In patients with acute neurologic conditions, there are specific issues and questions and several core competencies are required.

How can we best help families who are very frustrated with the situation and want to continue care against all odds? This chapter summarizes the main reasons and offers some approaches and solutions to resolve these cases outside the courts. In the United States, hospitals have been required by the Joint Commission to have medical ethics committees. When a discrepancy or conflict arises between a family and a physician, hospital ethics committees are usually asked to resolve the issue. Nonetheless, in many instances, significant frustration remains.[21,23,25,26]

The Ethical Dilemmas

Families are overwhelmed, grieving, and trying to come to grips with the acute situation. In other situations families are exhausted, do not know what to do, and see glimmers of hope all the time. When these glimmers seem to fade, something changes that motivates them to keep going on.

The main dynamics that maintain intransigence should be discussed here. First, the difficulty with prognostication has been touched on in prior chapters of this book, but can be briefly summarized as follows. One major reason not to withdraw medical support for some family members is their perception that outcome is inherently unknowable. These family members have noted uncertainty and more generally are convinced that no physician can be indubitably right. In their opinion, all prediction is uncertain, and even if there is, let's say, a 90% chance of poor outcome, there is still a 10% chance of good outcome. Many cannot believe physicians even have the capability of predicting a 99% probability of poor outcome.

Second, any respectful relationship between physician and family members requires recognition of cultural sensitivity. Failure to recognize that can quickly turn a cordial relationship into an embarrassment. In an increasingly diverse country, some groups of people may have a completely different view of how communication should proceed. In most of these cultures, there is simply a strong sense of obligation to their family member and to do all that is possible. In Asian cultures, nondisclosure is quite common. Discussion of the details of serious illness is often perceived as confrontational, disrespectful, taking away all hope, causing too much anxiety to the patient and even serious depression. Directness is often seen as cruel to the patient and as doing more harm—which of course it is not. The elderly are highly respected and revered, and their vulnerability might be undermined with such an approach.

Occasionally there are concerns raised by certain ethnic groups. Some African Americans have a continuous distrust of white physicians stemming from earlier days of humiliating segregation, and some assume that there is some element of discrimination in any type of health care. In the case of Latin Americans, lack of knowledge of their language increases the risk of conflict.[16]

Third, religious values are quite prevalent that emphasize life has value even if there is suffering. The Catholic Church has always advocated supporting life in devastating illness but also supporting suffering families. It is undoubtedly true that religious and cultural perspectives play a major role in the decision of families not to withdraw support. On balance, physicians respect all faiths, and their only task is to say words of comfort and express understanding. Paradoxically, most people of faith do understand and accept the legitimacy of stopping unnecessary treatment. Religious leaders of various denominations can often help clarify misbeliefs a person might hold regarding their church traditions and termination of care. They are crucial in helping to bring families closure by relieving their guilt related to their religious beliefs.

Another common issue is belief in divine intervention that supersedes biological certainty. Many Americans do believe in miracles. God may work his ways through physicians. Unexpected recovery is different from a miracle and obviously may occur. Believing in miracles undoubtedly impacts care, obviates do-not-resuscitate orders, reduces measures to de-escalate care, and may even increase level of care—there may be no end to last-resort measures.[6]

Of course, one major aspect in all of this is dealing with the suffering of the patient. Examples are the paralyzed ALS patient on mechanical ventilation, the debilitated stroke patient, and, in less obvious forms, the patient cognitively impaired as a result of destructive encephalitis. Many Christians and Asian cultures do emphasize sacrificing their lives to care for the disabled.

Another aspect that may come into play is that the central tenet of the major religious traditions has been the expectation of an afterlife. There can be two sides to this in end-of-life contexts. Major unexpected neurologic illness may be seen as punishment from God, and judgment after death may follow. On the other hand, concepts of paradise (from the old Persian word *pairadaeza*, meaning royal park or garden) with images of fields may be held, in which case the thought of patient and family being reunited later may help in finding closure.

More complex beliefs may be illustrated by traditional Hinduism, where—through the concept of karma—patients get what they deserve, and Japanese Shinto rituals that emphasize appeasement of the restless souls of the dead. Complex Chinese and Japanese beliefs and customs may interfere with adequate pain management. Buddhism addresses the importance of relief of pain as long as it does not cause significant sedation. Buddhists may accept death more easily than pain. Causing oneself pain is known in some religious groups and is considered a way of atoning for sins. It is easy to see how such reasoning can be an impediment in moving forward with providing the medically most appropriate level of care.

Fourth, failure to achieve closure may have its source in interpersonal conflicts. Conflicts may be between families and the attending physicians, within the attending physicians' team, or between family members.[1,3,4,8] Such a conflict is a significant threat not only to quality of care but also to what essentially must be a cordial relationship. Not well known and not often mentioned is that conflict within the healthcare team may be a source of concern. Different opinions or personal biases of the healthcare providers, crossing boundaries and becoming the family's advocate, or even worse, simply being oblivious to the true seriousness of the disorder—all of these may lead to inaccurately hopeful statements to the family members, followed by more confusion. Conflicts within the team itself—between nurses and physicians or physicians and residents—can all lead to persons feeling that their input or insights are not sufficiently valued. Nurses may feel that their continuous presence with the patient is not appreciated.[11] Physicians should also recognize that—in any system with shift schedules—attitudes of physicians may change and a new physician with the good intent to "solve this problem" may suddenly confront family members and confuse them even more.

A family conference cannot proceed unless the leading physician and nursing staff have a similar concept of what is happening to the patient and what the level of care should be. A conversation with the family cannot proceed if the healthcare providers are not "on the same page."

Conflicts may also be present inside a family structure. Different opinions will likely create the inability to make important decisions. Most of the conversation may have to do with straightening out these conflicts rather than discussing the wishes of the patient. These disagreements should be recognized. The overwhelming majority of other conflicts, however, are between clinicians and family members.[27] In order to manage conflicts between physicians and families, some skills are needed. First, any physician who encounters these situations will have to continue to display fair-mindedness and prudence and maintain professional integrity. This requires an inordinate amount of time and often multiple meetings with family members to come to a conclusion.[6,9,10,14,15,18,19,20] Second, a physician with good communication skills should be sought to help all healthcare workers to participate in a family conference. There should be clear reassurance to the family that the patient's cultural attitudes are valued. Barriers to communication, including family dynamics, should be identified very early. Conflict resolution can sometimes be achieved only after greater-than-normal time spent explaining the plan and expectations to the family. The consequences of a conflict not only impact patient safety and quality of care but also can lead to progressive mistrust, dissatisfaction, burnout, and misunderstanding with staff, as well as increased healthcare expenditure due to increase length of stay.

From a family point of view, conflicts are typically related to unsatisfactory communication with no follow-up on requests for information, professional staff behaviors that—in their view—include disrespectful or dismissive attitudes, families' perception that there is a time pressure on them to make a decision, and sometimes even nursing care causing the patient pain.[13] Many of these factors undermine confidence in the trustworthiness of physicians and nurses.

One solution was suggested by the San Francisco Bay Area Network of Ethics Committees. This procedure included consultation with a second physician who could approach the family and seek agreement. If no agreement was reached, the primary physician would present the case to a hospital ethics committee. If the committee disagreed with the primary physician, the patient was considered for transfer to another physician or another institution. If there was an agreement between the committee and the primary physician, the family was advised to seek a court order to continue treatment or request that the family member be transferred to a physician at another hospital. If transfer could not be arranged, withholding and withdrawal of nonbeneficial treatment would be considered ethically feasible. However it is unclear whether such a procedure would lead to resolution of continued futile treatment.[23]

Another core principle in discussion with the family is to try to define "futility." Historically, futility assessment did drive prognosticating scoring systems, including the APACHE score that could define poor outcome in intensive care patients and also identify whether high costs would be necessary to treat them. Some of this is also driven by the shortage of ICU beds and hospital administrators asking physicians to use these beds sparingly and wisely.

Futility can be loosely defined as inability to accomplish a treatment goal. Others prefer the term "potentially inappropriate."[28] In acute neurologic conditions this can be fairly simply defined as an inability to recover from unconsciousness or inability to become independent of intensive neurocritical care or medical care.[22,24] Futility implies that it is highly unlikely that patients survive their acute neurologic injury even with aggressive neurocritical care. This includes all patients who are facing imminent death due to a fatal, untreatable, unsurvivable disorder and typically includes patients who are comatose with additional brainstem injury and absent motor response or only reflex motor movements.

There are more problems with the term "futility." There simply might be lack of agreement on what constitutes beneficial treatment to the patient. In addition, there is a concern that physicians may not accurately present prognostic estimates. It is well known that nonspecialist physicians overestimate poor outcomes and underestimate good outcomes, particularly on the first hospital day. A recent study in the neurologic intensive care unit found that neurointensivists achieved reasonable accuracy in predicting functional outcome in patients with severe acute brain injury and had better accuracy in predicting poor outcome than good outcome.[12]

In Practice

In the vast majority of cases, failure to proceed with terminal neuropalliation is caused by (1) physicians not providing the information needed to make an informed decision; (2) pro-life cultural attitude or religious obligations that prevent patients' families from withdrawing support; (3) distrust, anger, and other emotions clouding medical reality; (4) families fearful of later remorse and (5) hope for propitious circumstances (6) a combination of all of the above or simply uncontrollable irrational behavior. Families might be unhappy with how patients have been treated, and in most instances, there is simply a sense of dissatisfaction among family members with the provided care when the patient is facing medical problems that might not seem so insurmountable to them ("not everything has been done").[5,7] Some family members do not accept the inevitable mortality of a loved one. Some families do not accept the limits of medicine. Some maybe be driven by unresolved conflict and can't make the decision to stop. This may lead to an extremely powerful defense mechanism and continuous requests for treatment.

In a particular family, decisions might be put forward by several members in the group. They may express the need to "fight" also, because they see their loved one as a "fighter." There is a general sense in these family members that one is able to "fight" a disease. Major medical diseases are seen as battles that have to be won and, in fact, can be won if only there is sufficient willpower to do so. Such family members have decided that a long-suffering road should be accepted and they therefore will have to face the reality of multiple complications, multiple interventions and, most of all, multiple discomforts to the patient. (I have seen an example of a patient with metastatic melanoma with multiple cerebral hemorrhages and multiple admissions for seizures including mechanical ventilation for status epilepticus until, finally, the family members decided to withdraw support.)

The conversation with some families may quickly turn awkward if family members, after a detailed explanation of the expected outcome, retort, "Yes, but stroke victims can improve, and he does not give up easily." Other family members cannot grasp the clinical context and are just flustered by the whole situation. They suggest that decisions will be made, but when asked, they do not truly want to make a decision. They always lean toward palliative care but never come to it. In these situations, the physician and family relationship can also become markedly tense.

How can we bring closure to these difficult situations? Table 10.1 summarizes some of the necessities before level of care is discussed. This requires multiple, scheduled, prolonged family conferences consistently bringing a message that summarizes the medical condition. Families should hear, every day, that there is no hope for improvement and that the medical conditions will only get worse. Clarification remains important, if not the most crucial element in resolving conflict, and this includes the explanation of different comatose states. Opening of eyes, blinking, grimacing, grinding of teeth, and sleep-wake cycles could be part of a developing vegetative state, and these manifestations should be explained as unpurposeful. In these conversations, the level of care should be clearly spelled out, and deadlines should ideally be set. For example, a do-not-resuscitate order should be followed by withdrawal of antibiotics, followed by removal of the

Table 10.1 **How to Prepare for a Difficult Family Conference**

- Have the latest medical information.
- Have nursing staff available.
- Ask family members to summarize their understanding of the bigger picture.
- Ask family members what would constitute futility in their minds.
- Acknowledge their hope.
- Avoid defensive behavior.
- Maintain a lead and avoid "sidelining."
- Acknowledge a willingness to be self-critical and that prediction is complex.
- Acknowledge adaptability and that the situation may change.

ventilator. Removing all intervention at once is often seen as "pulling the plug" and may be poorly handled by family members. In addition, one should try to identify the so-called obstructive factor that interferes with withdrawal of support. It is not inappropriate to gently confront family members regarding what their goal of care is, what they expect, and what obstructs letting go.

If a surrogate decision-maker (usually the spouse or another close family member) is not acting in the best interest of the patient, a court-ordered change can be sought. This would place such a case in a much different light and lead to far more frustration, but sometimes there is no other way. Nonetheless, some bioethicists see "little hope for medical futility"[7] as a result of courts yielding to "autonomy over professional determination of futility."

In summary, three main steps have been recently been suggested to change the climate of continuous care. First, physicians should be more measured in their enthusiasm regarding whether the patient could eventually recover, and should try to avoid false hope. Second, clear limits should be established once a major intervention is undertaken. When there is no benefit, there should be no continuation of aggressive care. Third, physicians should be willing to sincerely voice their best assessment rather than leaving patients' families in the dark. Vague descriptions of the medical condition to family members could lead to high expectations and failure to cope with disappointment. It remains to be seen—and tested—where effective communication may avoid disputes or whether a mediator seeking agreement helps in resolving disputes in patients with neuro-catastrophes. Finding another institution to care for the patient remains a very unsatisfactory resolution of a conflict.

In the United States, more than two-thirds of the states uphold the rights to withdraw artificial hydration and nutrition in a persistent vegetative state (PVS). The US statutes differ in their wording in three ways, with some referring to PVS, some to unconsciousness alone, and others to a terminal condition. Withdrawal of nutrition and hydration is not allowed in the United Kingdom and several countries in the European Union without a court order and is not an option in most

Asian countries. There always have been questions about how much courts should be involved in influencing medical decision-making at the end of life. Most physicians and attorneys see it as undesirable, and many supreme courts refuse to hear cases. Courts have always confirmed the rights of incompetent and competent individuals to receive or refuse treatment and have looked at the patients' "best interest." Some have argued that the mere fact that courts are there to potentially hear a case may paradoxically increase resolution of conflicts in the hospital setting.[29]

Many legal cases are settled in court without much attention. When a case comes to trial, there may be unforeseen consequences. It may lead to evaluation of professional standards of knowledge and an attack on the physician's credibility, whether the physician acted intentionally or even recklessly or displayed arrogance. Courts will look for experts to seek errors made in assessment and may even eventually impose sanctions on the physician or hospitals for misconduct.

Some a cases settled in court reach media attention. Unfortunately, these legal cases are surrounded by misinformation, politics, and sloganeering. In the United States, several landmark court cases are on record—all involved cases where everything that could go wrong went wrong. Disagreements not only involved physicians but often family members, with serious accusations. The attorneys often magnified the differences.

Finally, even situations may occur where the family does not accept brain death as death. For them, circulatory arrest is the only criterion. If families fail to accept brain death as death, there are two options. First, the physician could consider maintaining full support for 2–3 days while trying to resolve this issue and, in turn, ask for assistance from a hospital ethics committee to explain to the family that brain death is, in fact, the death of a person. Spiritual counsel may be sought. Physicians should appreciate these sensitivities and try to help family members achieve a sense of closure. Continuing support should be full support, and it is poor practice to maintain mechanical ventilation and stop vasopressors, effectively hastening cardiac arrest (cardiopulmonary resuscitation is not warranted under any circumstances). If the family refuses to come to an agreement and remains intransigent, legal advice should be obtained. A local judge will then decide and can be expected to declare the patient dead, which would then allow withdrawal of support. However as alluded to, once the issue is in court (and possibly several courts) a quick resolution cannot be expected. Moreover families may have a right to appeal a decision and a judge can order a restraining order preventing withdrawal of support pending appeal.

Later guilt (or remorse) is a powerful, anxiety-laden emotion (Table 10.2). It may come soon after the decision to withdraw has been made and may be disguised as anger. Most of these early emotions subside and reality sets in, but I have seen family members years after withdrawal of support question their actions even when the decisions at that time were made in the setting of overwhelming futility. Guilt in this context is also partly related to revisiting the physician's

Table 10.2 **Questions Families May Ask Later**

- Why has this happened?
- What can still be could have been tried?
- Was no stone left unturned?
- Was there pain perception?
- Was death peaceful?
- Was there starvation?

medical knowledge ("did he know the right things?") and revisiting their own decisions ("did I truly understand what I was told?"). Bereavement support should be sought, and ideally healthcare professionals should find ways to follow up by phone or e-mail if problems are anticipated. In some instances, repeating in a letter that "nothing could have been done" may bring closure. Physicians may need to appreciate that support may be needed for some time and follow-up phone calls in complex situations may help families to cope with loss.

Putting It All Together

- Denial is a common response and may persist
- The main reason for failure to grasp the seriousness of the clinical situation is often a "perfect storm" of unfamiliarity, strong personal values, and distrust of physicians
- Conflict resolution is possible in the majority of disputes, and bringing in a third party via an ethics consult is potentially helpful
- Cultural values are frequently misunderstood
- Involvement of courts should be avoided

References

1. American Society for Bioethics and Humanities. Core competencies for health care ethics consultation: the report of the American Society for Bioethics and Humanities. Glenview, IL. American Society for Bioethics and Humanities;1998.
2. Azoulay E, Pochard F, Chevret S, et al. Meeting the needs of intensive care unit patient families: a multicenter study. *Am J Respir Crit Care Med* 2001;163:135–139.
3. Azoulay E, Sprung CL. Family-physician interactions in the intensive care unit. *Crit Care Med* 2004;32:2323–2328.
4. Bloche MG. Managing conflict at the end of life. *N Engl J Med* 2005;352:2371–2373.
5. Boyd EA, Lo B, Evans LR, et al. "It's not just what the doctor tells me": factors that influence surrogate decision-makers' perceptions of prognosis. *Crit Care Med* 2010;38:1270–1275.
6. Bülow HH, Sprung CL, Baras M, et al. Are religion and religiosity important to end of life decisions and patient autonomy in the ICU? The Ethicatt study. *Intensive Care Med* 2012;38:1126–1133.

7. Caplan AL. Little hope for medical futility. *Mayo Clin Proc* 2012;87:1040–1041.
8. Cohen S, Sprung C, Sjokvist P, et al. Communication of end-of-life decisions in European intensive care units. *Intensive Care Med* 2005;31:1215–1221.
9. Culver C, Clouser K, Gert B, et al. Basic curricular goals in medical ethics. *N Engl J Med* 1985;312:253–256.
10. Cusveller B. Nurses serving on clinical ethics committees: a qualitative exploration of a competency profile. *Nurs Ethics* 2012;19:431–442.
11. Fassier T, Azoulay E. Conflicts and communication gaps in the intensive care unit. *Curr Opin Crit Care* 2010;16:654–665.
12. Finley Caulfield A, Gabler L, Lansberg MG, et al. Outcome prediction in mechanically ventilated neurologic patients by junior neurointensivists. *Neurology* 2010;74:1096–1101.
13. Fins JJ, Solomon MZ. Communication in intensive care settings: the challenge of futility disputes. *Crit Care Med* 2001;29:N10–N15.
14. Fletcher JC, Siegler M. What are the goals of ethics consultation? A consensus statement. *J Clin Ethics* 1996;7:122–126.
15. Helft P, Eckles R, Torbeck L. Ethics education in surgery residency programs: a review of the literature. *J Surg Educ* 2009;66:35–42.
16. Høye S, Severinsson E. Professional and cultural conflicts for intensive care nurses. *J Adv Nurs* 2010;66:858–867.
17. Keller B. How to die. *New York Times* editorial, 2012 Oct 7.
18. Larcher V, Slowther AM, Watson AR; UK Clinical Ethics Network. Core competencies for clinical ethics committees. *Clin Med* 2010;10:30–33.
19. Lilly CM, De Meo DL, Sonna LA, et al. An intensive communication intervention for the critically ill. *Am J Med* 2000;109:469–475.
20. Luce JM. A history of resolving conflicts over end-of-life care in intensive care units in the United States. *Crit Care Med* 2010;38:1623–1629.
21. Moeller JR, Albanese TH, Garchar K, et al. Functions and outcomes of a clinical medical ethics committee: a review of 100 consults. *HEC Forum* 2012;24:99–114.
22. Rabinstein AA, Hemphill JC, 3rd. Prognosticating after severe acute brain disease: science, art, and biases. *Neurology* 2010;74:1086–1087.
23. Rivera S, Kim D, Garone S, Morgenstern L, Mohsenifar Z. Motivating factors in futile clinical interventions. *Chest* 2001;119:1944–1947.
24. Rocker G, Cook D, Sjokvist P, et al. Clinician predictions of intensive care unit mortality. *Crit Care Med* 2004;32:1149–1154.
25. Schneiderman LJ. Ethics consultation in the intensive care unit. *Curr Opin Crit Care* 2005;11:600–604.
26. Schneiderman LJ, Gilmer T, Teetzel HD, et al. Dissatisfaction with ethics consultations: the Anna Karenina principle. *Camb Q Healthc Ethics* 2006;15:101–106.
27. Studdert DM, Mello MM, Burns JP, et al. Conflict in the care of patients with prolonged stay in the ICU: types, sources, and predictors. *Intensive Care Med* 2003;29:1489–1497.
28. Truog RD, White DB. Futile treatments in intensive care units. *JAMA Intern Med* 2013;173:1894–1895.
29. White DB, Pope TM. The courts, futility, and the ends of medicine. *JAMA* 2012;307:151–152.

Index

Page numbers followed by 'f' refer to figures.